# FORMULA 50

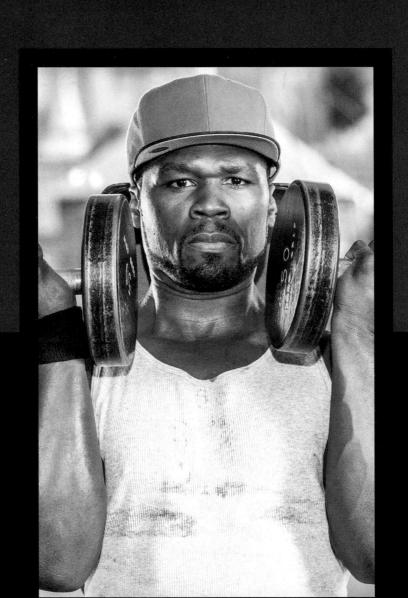

# FORMULA 50

## A 6-Week Workout and Nutrition Plan That Will Transform Your Life

## 50 CENT

with Jeff O'Connell

AVERY
a member of Penguin Group (USA)
New York

Published by the Penguin Group
Penguin Group (USA) LLC
375 Hudson Street
New York, New York 10014

USA · Canada · UK · Ireland · Australia
New Zealand · India · South Africa · China

penguin.com
A Penguin Random House Company

First trade paperback edition 2013
Copyright © 2013 by G-Unit Books
Photographs by Pavel Ythjall
Penguin supports copyright. Copyright fuels creativity, encourages diverse voices,
promotes free speech, and creates a vibrant culture. Thank you for buying an authorized
edition of this book and for complying with copyright laws by not reproducing, scanning,
or distributing any part of it in any form without permission. You are supporting writers
and allowing Penguin to continue to publish books for every reader.

Most Avery books are available at special quantity discounts for bulk purchase for
sales promotions, premiums, fund-raising, and educational needs. Special books or book excerpts
also can be created to fit specific needs. For details, write
Special.Markets@us.penguingroup.com.

The Library of Congress has catalogued the hardcover edition as follows:

50 Cent (Musician)
Formula 50 : a 6-week workout and nutrition plan that will transform
your life / 50 Cent with Jeff O'Connell.
p.        cm.
ISBN 978-1-58333-502-4
1. Physical fitness.   2. Exercise.   3. Weight loss.   4. Nutrition.
I. O'Connell, Jeff, 1963–   II. Title.
GV481 A126     2012              2012037786
613.7—dc23

ISBN 978-1-58333-532-1 (paperback edition)

Printed in the United States of America
1   3   5   7   9   10   8   6   4   2

Book design by Tanya Maiboroda

For Chris Lighty

# Contents

# 1

# Introduction

I DROPPED A LOT OF WEIGHT IN 2010, WHEN I TOOK A ROLE in a movie called *All Things Fall Apart*, playing the part of a cancer-stricken football player who would lose 60 pounds because of his illness. Scaling down from my usual 215 would mean running 15 miles not once but twice a day and surviving on a liquid diet for 10 weeks. Folks in my inner circle said I was crazy. They know I love to eat and didn't want to have to deal with me hungry. But sometimes you just have to challenge yourself.

Folks who know me best call me "The Machine." I may have gained fame singing about sipping Bacardi and hanging out in the club but, truthfully, my greatest vice is overwork. I go hard all the time and thrive off being strong, being successful, being fit, and ultimately being the best version of Curtis Jackson that I can be. Why? Coming up hard the way I did, I used to equate success purely with dollars. After *Get Rich or Die Tryin'*, I bought Mike Tyson's house in Connecticut on the spot. That was my confirmation of success. I walked into the house and was like: *I can buy this?* I wanted it not because I needed it, but because I could have it. So I moved out of a room in a basement to a 55,000-square-foot mansion with swimming pools.

I still get a rush off money, but I now realize it can serve a higher purpose: helping others. But unless you are physically strong and mentally tough, you can't go out and make that money to enjoy it with the ones you love, or for whatever purpose you have in mind. Besides, I just love winning.

In *The 50th Law*, which I wrote with Robert Greene, I taught readers the ten laws of strategy and success. Those laws have made me who I am today. Ultimately, the message boiled down to my essential creed: "Fear Nothing." The book sold well, but I am even prouder of how it changed lives. I decided that every book I write should do the same—change people's lives in some way. That's certainly true of the book you're reading now.

*Formula 50* builds on *The 50th Law* with an ambitious 6-week mind-body plan that can transform anyone serious about shaping up. My music, acting, business, and philanthropy cross all boundaries and barriers, and my fitness program applies to everyone too. All of you will see some version of yourself in this book. Not only your current self but the person you hope to become.

The basic 6-week plan targets beginners. Those with more workout experience under their belt can do the more advanced 6-week plan. Ideally, you'll progress through both plans over the course of 12 weeks, ending up where I am today with my fitness and body—good enough to hang with the world's best boxer, Floyd Mayweather Jr., during his training for championship bouts. I'm not promising that you'll be able to train with Floyd, but follow the instructions I'm giving you here, and you'll not only look a lot better but feel a *whole* lot better too. You'll be ready for whatever challenge life throws your way.

Fat, you don't stand a chance against Formula 50. Trust me, it's fire.

You might legitimately ask, "Who are you to preach about fitness? Aren't you the guy who dropped joints like 'High All The Time'? Hardly seems like a fitness anthem." I don't drink and I don't use drugs, and I didn't back then either. I put that joint on the first record because I saw artists consistently selling 500,000 with that content. Styles P, "Good Times (I Get High)"—that was on his gold album. Method Man and Redman were selling the same stuff. There was an audience that would accept it because they were actually high when *they* were listening to it. Plus, everyone was getting high around me, and that was actually what helped me decide not to. So I set off on a different course, one that depended on physical strength and fitness as well as inner strength and business smarts.

Today's up-and-comers do the same thing. I hear 'em mentioning Bentleys and Rolls-Royces and Ferraris and Lamborghinis. Well, *I'm* just getting to a point now where I can have those things with no problem. So they're lying. They don't have them. They have these bracelets and these rings but them diamonds ain't real in there. That's fake shit on 'em. It takes time for someone to reach that point.

Here, you're after something that's much more valuable than bling, fake or real. My point is that real results won't come easy; you need to put in the time and the effort, just like with anything worth doing. But in defining your body, you will develop a much clearer picture of what you're made of inside.

## Cutting-Edge Fitness That Works

My music is collaborative, and so was my approach to *Formula 50*. In deciding to write a fitness book, I obviously based it on my own extensive experience with working out. Only that wasn't good enough. I put the best minds in the health, fitness, and motivation world on the case. I wanted a program that would work for everyone and that everyone would want to follow. The perfect plan poorly executed or left on the shelf is worse than the average plan perfectly executed. It can be the most brilliant regimen in the world, one so effective that everyone doing it would be walking down the street with six-packs. Yet if only 50 percent or 10 percent of the people stick with it, I consider that program to be a failure.

The first rule of fitness is this: Show up for the workout. The workouts in *Formula 50* represent the cutting edge of exercise science and nutrition, but they're no good if you don't follow them. I don't want you to read this book; I want you to *use* it!

The reverse is true as well. Some so-called experts amp you up to such a degree that you're ready to run through a brick wall, only they never deliver a plan that will get you through to the other side. That's cold. You've gotten people to buy in and work out, but the tools you gave them weren't up to the job. What a letdown.

Formula 50 is a detailed workout and nutrition plan that will guide your fitness efforts over the course of 6 life-changing weeks. The carefully chosen array of exercises and meals form the foundation, but Formula 50 is about more than that. It's about learning how to become mentally as well as physically strong. You can never be happy with the workout you just had. If you can't outdo yesterday, you won't be better tomorrow.

These are the same tactics I use every day in my personal life. Fans know they work. My inner strength is rooted in surviving a spray of nine bullets to my face and legs, only to rebuild my body and mind into a superior force. Almost 120 million folks watched my "In Da Club" video on YouTube. The bat crunches I did with Dre and Eminem became one of the most iconic images in rap. Suddenly, everyone was eager for my methods: *How can I look like 50 Cent did in that video?* They've caught glimpses before, but never the full plan.

You're holding the plan in your hands: Formula 50. I'm now rich and famous, but I still go harder than the next guy, whether on stage, in the boardroom, or in the gym. I never coast, only accelerate. You have it within you to do the same. This is your guidebook.

## The Formula 50 Plan

So here is the promise I'm making: Follow my Formula 50 program, and your body will improve by 50 percent in 6 weeks. Body fat will decrease by 10 percent, energy will increase by 20 percent, and strength endurance will improve by 20 percent. The numbers can add up to 50 percent in a variety of ways, but your gains will total at least 50 percent. Fifty by 50.

Why are these measures so important, considering all the measures of fitness out there? Let me start by saying that there are dozens of ways to measure "fitness." There's power—that can be measured by your vertical or long jump. Flexibility can be tested by a straight-leg hamstring test. Cardiovascular fitness can be measured by comparing the difference in your resting heart from the beginning to the end of the 6 weeks.

You'll improve on every one of these tests over the course of Formula 50.

Having said that, I figure that virtually everyone who picks up this book will want to do three things: (1) drop some body fat, (2) have more energy, and (3) become stronger in the way that matters most—muscle endurance rather than brute strength. You may not care what you can lift for one all-out repetition on the squat, but wouldn't you love to carry around your young child without feeling old and broken down? Or take grocery bags from the store to your car without feeling like you just did an Ironman?

Those percentages I mentioned aren't pulled from thin air. They're totally legit. I've crunched data with leading exercise physiologists to ensure that the program will deliver those results.

## Your Secret Weapon: MRT

So how are we going to accomplish all of these physical improvements at once? Through metabolic resistance training (MRT), a workout system that breaks down the barriers between weight training and cardio. It's the fastest way to go from out of shape to in shape. We're not talking days—but we're not talking many months either. We're talking weeks. But to reach that goal, there's no fooling around.

We're going to bump some major workouts on this program, designed by me and Joe Dowdell, CSCS. No yakking with your boys in between sets or grinding at one pace on the treadmill; nothing but heat. Rest periods separate many sets, but you'll need to spend them sucking down as much oxygen as possible. What's more, those rest periods often shrink from week to week, making the workouts progressively more challenging. The manipulation of rest periods is one of the keys to the program.

MRT burns fat at the same time it builds muscle and lung power. Instead of tapping 25 percent or 30 percent of the body's change capacity, you're maximizing its full potential. The metabolic forces unleashed work even while you sleep. Such round-the-clock improvement makes it possible to improve by 50 percent in 6 weeks. Better yet, you can shift those percentages depending on whether your personal target is more strength, energy, or fat loss. However, they'll still add up to 50.

These multiple goals make the plan unlike anything the mainstream fitness world has seen. It's fluid, it's flexible, and it allows you to shape it according to your own needs and goals. It focuses on the attributes that truly matter in life: leanness, strength, and energy. Abs come as a bonus or byproduct, but they come because you're doing everything else right, instead of wasting your time doing crunch after crunch. The abs symbolize something greater. There needs to be something more.

Previously, only elite coaches to high-level athletes applied the advanced training and nutrition concepts in Formula 50. My team and I aim to make these concepts understandable and accessible to everyone, allowing you to achieve optimal results from a transformation program. A basic plan will apply to beginners, as well as to those returning from a layoff. In each of these 6 weeks, you'll do MRT-style resistance training three times a week and cardio twice. But none of this simple back-on-this-day, chest-on-that day junk. No workout will focus on isolated body parts. Is that how you move, with just one arm, or just your lat muscles? That's old-school training and deserves to be stowed in the attic. Do you still dress like you did in the 1990s or dial a rotary telephone? So why do you still train that way?

A more advanced version of Formula 50—think of it as the remix—adds an additional day of energy system training, among other demands. This phase targets those of you already closer to my current fitness level. These are some serious workouts. You need to be in good shape already, or go through the first 6-week program if your fitness level trails where it should be.

Look, I'm at my peak, and yet I've been in the game long enough to show that my body and my career are both built to last. I wrote *Formula 50* for the same reason I produced a vitamin-water product and now seek to address hunger in Africa through Street King, an energy shot with a built-in charity component connected to the United Nations World Food Programme, aimed at providing 1 billion meals over the next 5 years. I want this program to fill the desperate need among people of all races and economic classes to retake control of their body through improved health and fitness. True power comes from sharing knowledge and opportunity, and we need more of both. "Before I Self Destruct" may have been the title of one of my recordings, but it shouldn't describe America's lack of fitness and overall health.

Too many workout programs leave people tired rather than energized, defeated rather than victorious, depressed rather than uplifted. Formula 50 isn't going to exhaust you; it's going to leave you amped by causing metabolic shifts that will burn through layers of fat and encourage muscle growth. I bring energy to everything I do, and if my body is the motor, my workouts are the fuel. Without them, I couldn't do what I do in any aspect of life.

6

Never is this truer than when I go on tour and play for crowds. Ninety minutes on stage means I have to train as if I'm preparing for a heavyweight fight, only there's no bell—the rounds just keep on going. Nonstop effort requires strength, endurance, flexibility, and mobility. My workouts are designed to improve all those capabilities.

Throughout this book, I'll be urging you to stay with me on this transformation journey. Your motivation may not be the same as mine. You may not have a concert tour coming up—but you might have a wedding or a high school reunion. Something in your life can motivate you to want to lose weight. I'll help you find your own transformation trigger, things you might want to try in your own life. There usually isn't just one, by the way; there might be ten that can be identified in each person. You just need a system for identifying them. I'll provide that.

Some fitness works devote a single chapter to the mind, but motivation drives Formula 50 from start to finish. I'll constantly help you quell the urge to quit. I've been there myself. I was the fat kid when I was younger! I know what that's like. Even today, I find myself in situations, like training with my buddy Floyd Mayweather, the world champion boxer, where he's kicking my butt all over the boxing gym. Can I keep up? For a while. Maybe. Am I getting an amazing workout even when I fade before Floyd? Of course. Someone can always train a little harder than you. Someone's genetic blueprint might be a little more ideal for fitness than yours, but that's just a random twist of DNA. What matters is what you do with it.

Your goal and my goal are one and the same: to become the best version of ourselves humanly possible. This whole process of working out and being fit carries great meaning for me. Sure, people who look fit are easy on the eyes, but my physical training gives me the discipline to conquer life's challenges. It gives me strength to apply leverage, power to influence, energy to execute. It elevates me while at the same time grounding me.

My entire career and life have been based on a series of principles. These include the importance of power, leverage, strength, and energy; the need to embrace change and chaos; and the foolishness of thinking you can succeed without a well-thought-out game plan. Even my workouts never occur at random.

From these principles come the laws I live by. Formula 50 will not only embody those laws but also create new ones that apply to working out and shaping up. These laws are designed to lead you down the shortest path to the best results. Through trial and error, and through meeting with leading experts in exercise science, I've figured out what works, and just as important, what doesn't work. You ready?

## Fifty's Laws of Fitness

### Law #1 Where there's a will, there's a way.

When people caught a glimpse of Internet images of me preparing for *All Things Fall Apart*, playing the part of an emaciated, cancer-stricken football player, rumors swirled that I was seriously ill or even dying. That's how quickly I lost weight doing marathon runs on a liquid diet. I needed to lose almost 60 pounds, and I did, because the role demanded that of me.

We tend to give up too quickly when it comes to working out and eating right. But in Formula 50, I don't complain about that tendency. It is what it is. I acknowledge it and offer a program and motivational support that allows you to succeed despite that tendency. I've interviewed a number of leading motivational experts and sports psychologists to pinpoint where and why people are most prone to trip up on transformation programs. Once you know the trouble spots, you can see them coming and have the last laugh when you blow past them.

### Law #2 Just because there's a way doesn't mean it's the best one.

It turns out that running 10 to 15 miles twice a day and starving yourself isn't the healthiest way to lose weight. Yes, it worked for me in that situation. But I could have done it more efficiently using circuit training and other forms of metabolic resistance training, high-intensity interval training (HIIT), and other techniques. That's what I do now. I still pour every ounce into my workouts, but I train smarter. I've even learned how to be stronger now than I was when I was bigger.

Formula 50 brings together leading exercise physiologists and nutritionists to present not only the best workout and diet plan but also the most efficient one. If everyone ran 30 miles a day, everyone would lose weight. Only no one would stick with it, so what would be the point? Not a good program. People buy in to what you're preaching and stay the course when they know you're offering them not a shortcut, necessarily, but the most direct way to transform.

## Law #3 Your most important muscle is your heart, so train it accordingly.

I'm gonna shine until my heart stops, like one of my best-known songs says, but I don't want it to stop for a long time, which means doing plenty of cardio. The heart is a muscle, and you want for it to be your strongest, best-conditioned muscle of all.

A hallmark of the Formula 50 program is that your body will improve according to many different measures, and not just those included in the formula. The ability of your heart and lungs to keep blood and oxygen flowing through your system will also improve dramatically after 6 weeks. In many respects, this is the best measure of all for "fitness." This sort of conditioning is also essential for long-term heart health, so the dividends keep on coming.

I'm particularly excited about bringing HIIT-style cardio to the masses. HIIT achieves better results than regular steady-state cardio and in much less time. Plus, it's a good acronym for any recording artist to hang his hat on, right?

## Law #4 Learn to embrace chaos in the gym. Turn it to your advantage.

Change is constant in Formula 50. You'll never do the same stuff for very long. Surprise your body and you can expect to achieve major results: more muscle and less fat. With my program, it works every time.

This has to be fun even when your brow is pouring sweat. On the Formula 50 program, you'll do weights one moment, interval cardio the next, and even the intervals can be done using almost any kind of technique or apparatus: sprinting, elliptical, bike, heavy bag, rower, hitting the mitts like I do with Floyd, power cleans, and so on. You'll be on your toes! Once the body grows accustomed to the same workout, which doesn't take long, the workout loses its effectiveness. Stagnation is bad. Change is good. Growth is better.

**Law #5** The gym is a place to build muscle and burn fat, not waste time.

The gym setting will produce the best results from training. If you're aiming to improve 50 percent in 6 weeks, you've got to be willing to go there for workouts. But the Formula 50 plan won't have you training in the gym for hours on end. Getting in and out means you can't take extended rest periods and joke around the whole time. The sort of metabolic shifts I already mentioned for fat burning and muscle building depend on you keeping rest periods tight. You need to enter the gym, do your weights and cardio efficiently, and then, boom, leave.

This efficiency reflects workouts that are dense and action-packed. They compress a lot of activity into relatively short stretches. As I explain how to use these techniques, I'll also share some of the research behind them. You're putting your faith (not to mention your body) in this program, and I hope you'll stay the course when you see it's legitimately supported by science.

## Fifty's Laws of Clean Eating

**Law #1** The best tat you can ever receive is a sculpted body, and if weights are the needle, your diet provides the ink.

You have to eat right to look good. There's a big difference between dieting and eating right. A lot of you who don't eat well may think of a diet as something exotic that they go on a certain number of days to produce a certain outcome. Instead, you should view healthy eating as something that can be followed lifelong for good health.

Formula 50 teaches healthy eating, not "dieting" in the short-term sense that it's often used. Pair your workouts with the right eating habits, and the gains will come fast. Fueled properly, the body can change, maybe not overnight, but in a matter of weeks. Realize that your optimum fuel mix may differ from mine, and from the next guy's or girl's too. Together, we'll figure out your ideal mix.

We know what works: Every man and woman who competes in a fitness or bodybuilding show follows some variation on certain parameters to shape up. You're probably not going to take your diet to the extreme that they do, but the same principles apply. In Formula 50, I make it all easy to understand.

**Law #2** Following the same old diet seldom works for a very long time because you get sick of the same old diet.

Your nutrition can benefit from change much like your workouts. Change keeps your head in the game. If you're being served chicken breasts and broccoli every day, your body might respond well. In fact, it probably will; those are great foods. But your mind will start to cave. At a certain point, you'll begin to cheat; eventually, your whole diet will collapse. So I look at the bigger picture, working with experts to fashion meal plans that satisfy not just your stomach and muscles but also your mind. So you'll keep right on following those meal plans.

Formula 50 won't provide a 1-day meal plan and then ask you to repeat it for weeks on end. The meal plans change just like the workouts.

**Law #3** Since my program is all about boosting your energy, finding your body's proper fuel mix is essential.

It turns out that you aren't what you eat—you are what your body does with what you eat. Because you're going to be kicking butt on the Formula 50 program, your body will have energy needs specific to not only working out but also working out according to my plan.

The Formula 50 nutrition plan is high in lean protein, is somewhat high in healthy fats, and contains moderate amounts of carbohydrates. But healthy carbs—not the kind you pull out of vending machines. We're setting an ambitious agenda for these 6 weeks, so you'll need to be popping when it come to your nutrition. Beast mode. Ultimately, results provide the best motivation. Just like when I'm recording an album, my madness has a method.

**Law #4** Skipping meals is just as bad as having too many cheat meals because one leads to the other.

In my line of work, I can spend a lot of time in rooms without windows, and the day can fly by so fast that I'll turn around and, bang, it's over. I can grow so wrapped up in my work that I even forget to eat when I should. I've come to realize just how unhealthy that is. After a work day spent without food, being famished makes you eat like an undisciplined crazy person instead of like someone sane and in control.

So I have to stay on the grind when it comes to eating and drinking like I should. Part of not skipping meals is following the detailed diet plan outlined in Formula 50. We're not going to be starving you here; you'll be guided to eat three to five meals a day, spacing them every 4 to 6 hours apart. My science team will explain why eating more frequently *doesn't* provide the metabolic boost purported by so many fitness coaches. It's an urban legend. In fact, the latest evidence suggests that eating a little less frequently may be more metabolically beneficial than eating more frequently. The reason you *should* eat up to five times a day is to feed your muscles. But don't do it to boost your metabolism.

**Law #5** I'm no angel, period, but that's especially true when it comes to my diet. I'll be doing this along with you and facing the same struggles and temptations.

They may call me "The Machine," but they don't call me "The Robot." I try not to eat pizza, candy, or cake. Still, sometimes I cheat. But I know the rules I'm supposed to follow, and the nutritional advice in Formula 50 is both cutting-edge and simple to follow. I'm sure you can identify with my occasional dietary lapses. Feel free to say, "Damn, you mess up too, Fifty? Okay, now I have something I can aim for that I can possibly achieve."

Formula 50 will include meal plans for the entire 6 weeks. These menus are varied, nutritious, and delicious. I'm known as a picky eater, and I like everything in this book. I'm betting these foods and these meals taste better than the vast majority of what you eat now. This has nothing to do with deprivation. You're going to be eating better than before.

You'll soon realize that training and eating Formula 50–style will give you the body you've always desired. For guys, the words you'll hear are *ripped, cut,* and *muscular.* Women will hear *sculpted, lean,* and *toned.* So given that both sexes will follow the same program—except for minor dietary differences, mostly in total calories—why do the results produce different looks?

One of the biggest misconceptions in fitness is that lifting weights and consuming protein with every meal will make guys look like he-men and women look like men.

Nothing could be further from the truth. When you lift weights and consume enough protein in tandem, muscle tissue grows and becomes stronger. At the same time, your body starts to lose fat. The latter can happen pretty fast; the former takes form gradually, with the rate depending on factors such as your sex, age, nutritional status, and genetics—the DNA that your mom and dad combined to make you.

When you lift and eat protein regularly, nature tends to reward you with what you want. The teenage guy gearing up for high school football season likely wants to put on muscle pretty fast, and he probably will. His hormones are primed to produce that effect. Testosterone is mostly a guy thing, and the younger the guy, the more T he will likely have. T also drives your libido. If you're a guy, I'm sure you remember what it was like to be a 17-year-old dude thinking about girls 24/7. Well, the same hormone that makes you girl-crazy also builds muscle.

This might surprise you, but the female body also contains testosterone—just not nearly as much as the bros. How big of a difference? Normal levels in men can range from 300 to 1,200 nanograms per deciliter (ng/dL); in women, those numbers fall into a range of 30 to 95 ng/dL. What the female body does contain in abundance are estrogens, a group of steroid hormones responsible for the development during puberty of female sex characteristics, such as breasts, and the growth and maintenance of the female reproductive system. Estrogens don't do much in the way of building muscle, however. Evolution hasn't designed women to need as much muscle as men do. The female body is designed to give birth and nurture offspring, not exert brute force in life-and-death situations like fighting and food procurement.

So how to explain female bodybuilders, those muscle women who work out a lot, eat plenty of protein, and seem to sport more muscle and deeper voices than many guys? Many of them take pharmaceutical versions of the hormones produced naturally in abundance by the fellas. Not only do these drugs help them build crazy muscle, but they also change other aspects of their physiology and appearance. These changes make them appear more male-like—hence their deep and husky voices and protruding Adam's apples.

None of these changes can emerge without those drugs. Training and diet simply don't produce this effect in women. On the contrary, the changes that happen naturally are feminine and make guys like me go, "Dayuuum!" when you walk by. The women turning up on fitness magazine covers and turning heads at the beach often lift weights and eat a lot like healthy guys, only in smaller amounts, reflecting their size. That's why you'll notice that the meals in Formula 50 differ more in quantity than type of food. In most cases, what's good for him is good for her, and vice versa. The same goes for the workouts. We're dealing here with universal laws of physics as they relate to flesh and bone, not gender. They apply equally to men and women. Repetitions will be the same for each; only the weight will differ.

Muscle doesn't look bulky; muscle looks hot. Muscle looks lean and fit and healthy. Even most of the girls who do figure or bikini contests usually lift hard and heavy, and they diet almost like bodybuilders. They just don't take the drugs or the excessive calories needed to gain that massive amount of muscle.

I'm not forgetting about you, guys. In some ways, you need Formula 50 most of all. My nutrition advisor for the book, Layne Norton, PhD, is a bodybuilder who trains physique athletes for contests, along with being an academic. He finds that men are more resistant to transforming than women. Says Layne: "Over half my clients are women, and in my experience, they're the ones more predisposed to taking action. Some men will say, 'Yeah, I don't like the way that I look, but it's not that big of a deal.' But there are very few women who are 40 pounds overweight who will say, 'You know, I'm comfortable with how I look. I'm good with this body.'"

If you aren't comfortable with how you look, or feel, or perform, Formula 50 is just what you need. Your transformation begins here and now. The next 6 weeks will change your life in ways you can't even imagine.

# 2

# 50 Reasons You Should Start Working Out Now

**Y**OU NEVER GET A SECOND CHANCE TO MAKE A FIRST impression, and when your first album release is the biggest hip-hop debut album, that's pretty cool. But what comes next? Along with being a successful musician and actor, I'm now a businessman running a diverse array of ventures that includes music ownership, artist management, film production, footwear and apparel, video games, publishing ventures, and health drinks and dietary supplements. I'm just getting started too. You haven't seen anything yet.

I approach business differently from other artists, though. Most of them sign an endorsement deal for a certain product, whereas I actually have become a principal in businesses such as Vitaminwater, Street King, and SMS Audio, which makes audio headphones that set the standard for high-quality sound. This approach seemed like the best way to build a fortune that would last. Now, of course, a lot of other artists are angling for those same kinds of opportunities. But The Kid planted the flag first.

I don't attach myself to these projects in name only; I also invest my time and hard-earned dollars. Like any good businessman, I expect a certain return on my investments. I've also come to look at health and fitness as an investment, one I make in myself. Reason #1) If you take even 30 of the 1,440 minutes in a day and use them to work out, your body will reap dividends for years to come. This keeps you healthy and active rather than sick or, worse, dead before your time. #2) Exercise can be your greatest ally as you charge your way through life. It has your back. Fitness can help you succeed in business, attract an amazing mate, avoid health problems, and feel content and fulfilled.

Too often the opposite happens. Bad habits (not exercising, eating too much, skipping sleep) take root instead of good habits. God forbid that at a certain point, your lack of fitness causes your heart to give way. You may not survive a heart attack, but if you do, exercise will become this delicate dance between helping your heart and putting it at risk. You'll need to exercise to prolong your life, but exertion will now challenge a damaged organ. If you think it's hard to work the treadmill when you're in top form, imagine having to follow a disciplined workout regimen knowing, in the back of your mind, that those same workouts could cause you great harm, up to and including death.

Better to understand the stakes now and take action, rather than lying in a bed in the ER, waiting for the results of an EKG and heart enzymes test to learn if you just had a heart attack. The harm done by that point can't be undone, and you'll live with it for the rest of your life, a life that won't be as long or as fulfilling as it should be.

Some people look at their kids and say, "I need to be a good role model for them. I also want to be around to watch them grow up." The best way to make sure that happens is by being fit and healthy. #3) No one can guarantee that you'll live to 100, but the odds shift in your favor when you train and eat right. #4) Even more important will be the quality of that longer life. You want to play with your kids when they're young, compete with them during their adolescence, and then enjoy the fruits of that effort when they become parents. At that point you want to be standing on the sidelines cheering them, not chair-bound and smiling meekly, the parents who can't lift their arms high enough to clap.

Here's an even more important consideration. #5) When deciding whether to work out and eat healthfully, your kids will take many of their cues from you. Only, not from what you say as much as what you do. Children will often turn a deaf ear to your words, but you can bet they'll mimic your actions. So if you're a smoker, and you tell your kid not to smoke, they'll often end up smoking. Many of today's smokers have parents who smoked. They inherited the bad habit. Fortunately, the same goes for a healthy habit. If you practice whatever you preach, your children are far more likely to copy you.

Often the reward for this sort of investment in your child's future is delayed. You'll hear parents say, "I used to go to the gym, and my son looked at me like I was crazy, before going back to his video games. However, he went away to college, and the next thing I know he's into working out and he comes home all buff." The child reaches a certain point when they are ready to do that. They don't want to be like Dad necessarily, but this is what they saw growing up, and your behavior influenced theirs.

My own son was 15 during the writing of this book. He was also my motivation for the book I wrote before this one, which was about playground bullying. I was relating a scenario to him because someone was being bullied at his school, and I was like, "Yo, but he probably did that because of *this*." I found myself relating the bully's perspective because I was a bully when I was younger. But having grown up, I understand that I was dealing incorrectly with my emotions. I had issues growing up. I lost my mom when I was 8 years old, and because of that I started hustling. I would associate everything good with my mom coming because she would always bring me presents. It was like, "Your mother's here, woo, light up, excited!" When your anchor is cut loose from your life, you can replace it with something good or something bad. I chose something bad, and I chose it because I didn't know any better.

Choosing to become fit in the face of life's adversity is being smart. #6) Fitness gives you a sense of control over your body and your life. It's not just the mind-set improvement; it's that you have more muscle, strength, energy, and drive. #7) Much of this is rooted in exercise- and diet-induced hormonal changes that occur, creating a positive feedback loop.

The feedback loop isn't merely an individual thing, though. My Street King energy shot is for those who are starving, sometimes to death, but a billion or so people worldwide now have the opposite problem: They consume more calories than they burn. The medical costs associated with chronic diet-based conditions like diabetes and obesity are skyrocketing. They threaten to bankrupt national health care systems worldwide. The tab for heart disease–related costs alone in the United States surpasses $100 billion a year. These projections, like the disease itself, are scary. We can't afford to pay the rising cost, in dollars or human suffering.

The solution is embracing an active lifestyle fueled by exercise and healthy eating. #8) I won't say exercise is like kryptonite against disease, but damn near. Heart disease, cancer, stroke, type 2 diabetes—virtually all of the leading causes of death in the United States have strong links to physical inactivity and poor diet. All you have to do to reduce your risk of developing any of them is eat right and exercise. The benefits become only more profound as you age.

Let me break down some of the major health problems that the workouts and meal plans in Formula 50 can help address. This list is by no means exhaustive:

*Alzheimer's disease.* #9) Exercise and diet may slow the progression of mind-erasing Alzheimer's disease. A study review on the effects of physical activity and Alzheimer's found that physical activity may improve cognitive function in older adults. Start now to raise your odds of never having to hear that horrible diagnosis.

*Back pain.* #10) Strengthening your core muscles and improving your flexibility and posture can help prevent or manage back pain, a problem that can make you miserable. When 46 obese adults suffering from low-back pain specifically followed a medically supervised diet and exercise program for a year, their pain lessened and they functioned better. Weight reduction was also associated with improvements in function.

*Heart disease.* #11) Regular exercise helps reduce risk of heart disease by strengthening your heart muscle, lowering blood pressure in those who already have high blood pressure, increasing "good" (aka HDL) cholesterol, lowering "bad" (aka LDL) cholesterol, and helping your blood flow where it needs to, uninterrupted. This is of upmost importance since heart disease is the leading cause of death in the United States, claiming more than 600,000 lives each year.

*Cancer.* #12) In a study of breast cancer patients, every 11-pound increase in weight increased cardiovascular and breast cancer mortality by 19 and 13 percent, respectively. #13) And, fellas, in a review of 40 epidemiological studies, 22 suggested that physical activity reduced the risk of prostate cancer. #14) Colon cancer has a direct correlation with physical activity independent of other health measures. Environment also plays a role, but the connection between lifestyle and cancer is unmistakable and isn't just about smoking (although that's terrible).

*Obesity.* This one seems obvious but bears repeating. #15) In a study of 1,621 Portuguese adults, the most active study participants had a 40 percent lower risk of becoming obese than those who were less active. Not surprisingly, the more physically active the participant, the lower his or her risk of developing obesity.

*Rheumatic diseases.* #16–18) Proper diet and weight loss have shown effectiveness in studies at alleviating gout, fibromyalgia, and rheumatoid arthritis. These are grueling diseases that stick you with chronic pain.

*Osteoporosis.* Your muscles aren't the sole beneficiaries of fitness; so are your bones. #19) Weight-bearing exercise (walking, jogging, stair climbing, weightlifting) helps strengthen bone formation while preventing bone loss.

*Stroke.* Exercise protects not just your body but your brain as well. #20) According to a study in the journal *Stroke*, moderately active study participants were less likely to suffer stroke than less active ones.

*Type 2 diabetes.* #21–22) Exercise can increase insulin sensitivity, improve blood sugar and cholesterol, and improve heart function, all of which are enormously beneficial for diabetics. #23) A study in the *Annals of Internal Medicine* showed that increased physical activity, including regular walking, can help reduce the risk of cardiovascular events in diabetic women.

#24) Intensive lifestyle intervention may help reduce cardiovascular risk factors in diabetics. In a study of 5,145 overweight or obese people with type 2 diabetes, those who received intensive lifestyle intervention maintained greater improvements in weight, fitness, blood sugar control, systolic blood pressure, and good cholesterol after 4 years than those who received the regular protocol regarding support and education.

#25) Big, positive diet change may help treat type 2 diabetes better than traditional diabetes meds do. Nearly 600 recently diagnosed type 2 diabetics were divided into three groups: One group received a standard initial dietary consultation and twice-yearly follow-ups; another received dietary consultation every 3 months as well as monthly nurse support; and a third group received the latter plus they followed a pedometer-based activity program. After a year, the two intervention groups saw greater improvements in blood sugar and insulin sensitivity than the control group did, despite using fewer diabetes drugs and in small doses.

This should give you some sense of the "health insurance" provided by daily exercise and smart food choices. Life comes with no guarantees, and your health is no exception. There's always going to be the healthy person who dies young and the smoker who grows old. They're statistical outliers. Just like in the entertainment business, sometimes you do everything right and things still turn out wrong. #26) Still, shift probabilities in your favor, and odds are you'll make out all right.

## Zzzz's By the Numbers

On the Formula 50 program, it's imperative to sleep long enough and well enough to gain maximum benefits from your hard training and clean eating. I'm talking 7 to 8 hours a night, at least most nights. That range seems to be a sweet spot for good health. The risk of health problems seems to rise when people sleep only 6 hours or 9 or more. Surprisingly, sleeping *too much* is also unhealthy. Rip Van Winkle didn't wake up ripped, that's for sure.

Getting enough sleep greatly raises the odds that you'll hit the gym for your workouts. When scientists evaluated the health of more than 8,000 Japanese men, those who banked at least 7 hours a night were the most likely to exercise regularly. In contrast, those who slept fewer than 5 hours had the most irregular exercise habits and a whole host of health problems to boot. Achieving proper sleep should be a major public health concern, the study's authors said.

Ladies, you aren't immune from this phenomenon either. In a study of 291 college girls in northern Taiwan, those with poor sleep quality were more likely to lack physical fitness, including muscular endurance, flexibility, and cardiovascular fitness. What makes for poor sleep quality? Short sleep duration, daytime sleepiness, and difficulty falling asleep in the first place.

#27) This works in reverse: In a study of about 3,000 adults ages 18 to 85, getting 150 minutes a week of moderate to vigorous exercise was linked to a 65 percent improvement in quality of sleep. Another study found that exercise improved the quality of sleep in elderly insomniacs when they followed a regular cardio routine for 4 months. They reported a better quality and longer duration of sleep than those who stayed on the couch. #28) They also experienced a decrease in depressive symptoms and daytime sleepiness, as well as a boost in vitality.

#29) Exercise may be beneficial in treating sleep apnea, even beyond its weight-loss effect. (Obesity may cause obstructive sleep apnea, so losing weight by any means tends to help.) In one study, overweight and obese adults were divided into two groups. One performed 150 minutes a week of moderate-intensity aerobic activity and resistance training twice a week. The other met twice a week for low-intensity stretching. After 3 months, the exercise group had less severe sleep apnea, even when the members weighed nearly the same.

Kids and adolescents sometimes think they're indestructible. They figure sleep is the last thing they need, and they act accordingly. The actual sleep need of a young adult has been estimated at 8.5 hours, yet only 14 percent of young adults report sleeping for 8.5 hours or more on weekdays.

#30) One study linked vigorous exercising to sounder sleep and psychological functioning in adolescents, especially the young bucks. #31) Scientists also connected dots between a) high perceived physical fitness and b) favorable scores for various sleep indicators among young adults, even when a disconnect developed between someone's perception of their fitness and how much they actually worked out. In other words, some of it might have been in their head, true. But what was in their head was positive energy.

I'm not saying that if you go out and party too much and miss a few nights of good sleep as a result, all is lost body- and health-wise. But poor sleep can knock you off this program in the short term and harm so many different aspects of your health over the long term. Did you know, for example, that not getting enough sleep might be a contributing factor to obesity, diabetes, and even cancer? That poor sleep increases your odds of having a heart attack or stroke? One likely reason is that blood pressure is designed to fall while we sleep. Interrupting this natural rhythm stresses the cardio-vascular system.

That's why people who do shift work and pull strange hours need to be especially careful. One study found that women working rotating night shifts are more likely to develop type 2 diabetes than women working standard 9-to-5 gigs. In another study, this one of almost 5,000 American and Canadian police officers, some 40 percent screened positive for at least one sleep disorder. Most of them had not been previously diagnosed. What's more, those who screened positive for a sleep disorder were more likely to make a serious screw-up, fall asleep at the wheel, or commit an error or safety violation attributed to fatigue. They were also more likely to exhibit uncontrolled anger toward suspects, be absent from work, and doze off during meetings.

One reason a lack of sleep wreaks havoc on mind and body is that while you're sleeping, many of your hormones are hard at work on your behalf. Guys, especially, need to be aware that testosterone and growth hormone are at their most active during sleep. If you're not sleeping enough, your endocrine system can't supply the rest of your body with a full natural dose of these hormones. In stark contrast, cortisol, one of the hormones that tends to interfere with both muscle growth and fat loss, rises as sleep falls.

Furthermore, sleep disorders often occur as "comorbids"—medical "partners in crime," if you will—with medical conditions such as chronic pain, dementia, and stomach problems. Call it a feedback loop, meaning sometimes the medical condition interrupts sleep, sometimes poor sleep causes or worsens the medical condition, and sometimes both happen at once. The negative health effects of sleep are so widespread in part because poor sleepers tend to be messed up in other ways. In one study, unhealthy behaviors such as smoking and being a couch potato were more prevalent among those who slept fewer than 6 hours compared with those who slept 7 or 8 hours.

Along with hurting your body, poor sleep also imperils your mind. People who suffer from sleep disorders may even be at increased risk of suicidal behavior. Poor sleep has predictable negative health consequences, but it's also an accident waiting to happen. What did the Exxon *Valdez* oil spill, Chernobyl, Three Mile Island, and the *Challenger* space shuttle explosion all have in common? Worker fatigue was cited as a factor in all of these disasters. Who knows how many people have died in traffic accidents because they were sleepy or dozed off.

I'm pounding away on this topic because sleep is one of the biggest limiting factors to your success on my program. These workouts are challenging, and it takes dietary discipline to transform. When you stay up too late, you wake up too late, miss breakfast, postpone your workouts, and things unravel. Your day begins the night before. Mess that up and you won't be as productive and fit as you could have been.

#32) Exercise benefits your mind and mood as much as it does your body. #33) Researchers have connected fitness to self-confidence and self-discipline. The amount of literature linking increased physical fitness with positive psychological outcomes was already substantial by 1999, when scientists at the University of Missouri–Columbia attempted to gauge both the short- and long-term psychological effects of aerobic exercise. After 12 weeks, a group of people who pedaled a stationary bike saw greater improvements in mood and fitness than non-exercisers. Seven months later, the bikers were still better off physically and mentally.

The psychological benefits of exercise aren't limited to adults either. #34) A study review of 23 randomized controlled trials suggests that exercise may have a positive short-term effect on self-esteem in kids and adolescents. My guess is that the long-term effects are even more powerful.

*Self-esteem* refers to an internal state but is often measured by how you present yourself. High self-esteem is associated with willingness to accept risks, focus on the positive, and call attention to one's self. Speaking of which, you want high self-esteem, but not so high that you're bordering on narcissistic. I see a lot of that fronting in the rap game, and it spells trouble.

In contrast, low self-esteem is associated with a tendency to present yourself in a self-protective way, like you're scared. You won't take risks and don't call attention your way. How we view ourselves seems to influence how we treat others. Those with high self-esteem tend to treat themselves and others well, while those with low self-esteem tend to treat themselves and others poorly.

So if we know that fitness leads to self-confidence, does that self-confidence lead to success and a sense of well-being and high self-worth? Think of it another way: Are people successful because they're self-confident, or are they self-confident because they're successful? I think it works both ways.

For me, #35) stress prevention and management are the most immediate mental benefits of working out. I have a lot going on at any one time, but I'm seldom in one place for very long. I'm writing this passage on a jet that took off from an airport in New Jersey, a short drive out of Manhattan, and is destined for Burbank in southern California; I'm accompanying Floyd Mayweather and his crew. We had just flown in to Jersey the night before, and we won't be in LA for long either. This is a snapshot of my daily life. I live in Connecticut, but I'm usually there for only 1 or 2 days a month. The rest of the time I'm traveling, whether it's for a tour, business, or to support a friend like Floyd.

#36) Exercise can anchor a high-flying lifestyle like mine, or a demanding one that involves no travel. It keeps you cool under any circumstance. #37) You feel better just because you're accomplishing something good for you. If you've been stressing about carrying a few extra pounds, not looking your best, well, those weights fly off your shoulders when you start lifting.

The stress-reduction effects go to the very core of your being. #38) When you exercise, your brain offers you a reward by releasing endorphins. These brain chemicals make you feel high naturally. Exercise habitually and you feel good all the time. If they could bottle endorphins and sell them legally, drug dealers would be out of business. The effect is that powerful.

#39) Training also focuses your mind on something other than what's stressing you out. If recording in the studio was a struggle that day, I can carry that with me, or I can go the gym and let it go. When I'm repping under a barbell, I don't have the luxury of worrying about not getting a track just right. I lock into the movement, the rhythm, and that becomes my immediate reality. #40) In that sense, it's like meditation in motion.

#41) Exercise also makes you sleep better, and better sleep helps manage stress. So as I explained earlier, make sure to get your eighty winks.

#42) Given that exercise prevents stress and boosts your mood, no surprise that working out tends to work against depression, the clinical state in which sadness and stress take over. #43) Resistance training and cardiovascular training work equally well at battling the blues, and my program combines both. The catch-22, of course, is that when you're depressed, you don't want to go to the gym, even though you know it's good for you. I'm here to encourage you and even kick your butt a little when needed, a little tough love, 50 Cent–style. The effects don't happen overnight. Studies seem to find a noticeable improvement after a month or so of training, with maximum benefits kicking in after several months.

While the majority of benefits relate to important things like fitness, energy, and health, #44) working out can also improve your physical appearance in undeniable ways. First off, #45) clothes just look better on you when you're in shape. #46) Broad shoulders tapering down to a narrow waist symbolizes strength and masculinity in guys, and women benefit equally from a sculpted V-taper. Other body parts also impart symbolic importance and power, but only if they're trained and developed. #47) For guys, strong forearms are essential if you're going to rock the kind of watches I wear.

You can't have that sort of bling hanging from a spindly stick. #48) Calves are important for the ladies anytime they wear high heels.

The strength and power you develop from my workouts will give you a certain gravitational pull as a person. Where I'm from, you have to meet aggression with aggression. If you don't have a problem with a problem, other people steer clear of you because it could lead to a mess. That's why you never want to even suggest that it's okay to test you in that way. If they know you'll respond, they won't bother provoking you.

So you need to become what I like to call the lion in the room. If the person in one chair is the lion in the room, no matter how interesting other people are, they don't warrant attention. Only the lion does. The lion doesn't even have to move. Just us knowing the lion's capabilities, what *could* happen, is enough. The lion has true power.

I was in a movie with Bruce Willis, and I spent a lot of time observing his demeanor. He'd whisper stuff like, "I'm really into this project; I think it will be good." I'd be like, "What the fuck are you saying, Bruce? I can't hear you."

He was controlling the room. He knows he's Bruce Willis. He knows he's number one. And while he's talking, everyone in the room is interested. They're leaning in like, *What is he saying?* Later, I asked him, "Why were you speaking so low like that, Bruce?" He was like, "I'm controlling the room." It's not often you see people conscious of it and doing it for that purpose.

The self-confidence needed to be lion in the room can be developed in various ways. Bruce had it because he had become an international movie star in *Die Hard* and other blockbuster films. #49) One way you can achieve your own lion status as a person is by training and getting in shape. #50) Formula 50 will allow you to achieve more by speaking less. You will have found the true sources of your inner strength and power: physical fitness and mental toughness.

# 3

# 10 Fears That Can Lead to Failure

NO ONE DISPUTES THAT THE UNITED STATES AS A whole is overweight and out of shape. America may be the land of the free and the home of the brave, but we're also the land of the couch and the home of the potato. More than one-third of our children are overweight or obese. That's not a very promising future.

At this point it's more about motivation and enlightenment. No one's like, "Oh, *exercise*? So that's good for my health? Fifty, man, never heard that one before!" There's no shortage of information and other resources. Books (like this one) are written, magazine articles published, diets promoted, transformation contests held. The diet book category alone on Amazon.com has 30,000 titles.

Yet, as a society, we're getting fatter rather than fitter.

Anything that encourages healthy transformations should itself be encouraged. We've all seen the before-and-after pics people snap, smart phone in one hand, newspaper in the other. Occasionally this is smoke and mirrors, but much more often than not, people are legitimately transforming.

Unfortunately, many people remain unmoved to take action. The couch wins. What's more, many who try these programs don't succeed. Of those who join a gym, between 30 and 40 percent don't renew their gym membership and presumably stop training. Many of those who do sign up again don't actually work out, or they keep going to the gym yet fail to achieve their desired results.

The fact that there are so many new programs every January tells you something isn't working. If everybody shaped up, that would be that.

People fail for any number of reasons, but it often boils down to them talking themselves out of a fit body, telling themselves they won't make it. The mind sabotages the body. If you say those things long enough to yourself, eventually you start believing your own BS.

When it comes to becoming healthy and fit, it's easy to think of reasons why you won't succeed. I can rattle off ten right now. Maybe you've heard or even uttered them.

**1** I don't have time to work out or prepare healthy meals.

**2** I tried it before, and it didn't work. Why should I try again?

**3** I don't have good genetics. I'm not going to look like a fitness model anyway.

**4** I don't live near a gym, and I couldn't afford one even if I did.

**5** Every time I talk about working out and losing weight, my family members—who are also overweight and out of shape—ridicule me for the idea.

**6** I'm so damn out of shape that I'll never be able to lose this weight.

**7** I don't know what to do in the gym. It seems intimidating to me.

**8** I'm not overweight, so I'm already in shape without training or adhering to a healthy eating plan.

**9** I don't want to be one of those people carrying Tupperware full of stinky fish into meetings at work. Ugh.

**10** My garage is full of fitness equipment I picked up on HSN and QVC. All it's doing is collecting dust. That's proof that I can't do this!

Okay, let's go through these Frequently Mentioned Excuses (FME) one by one:

## 1. I don't have time to work out or prepare healthy meals.

Each day contains 24 hours, and working out and eating healthfully take only a very small percentage of that time. So, by definition, you have time for fitness.

What you're really saying is that other activities take precedence over your health. On your list of priorities, health-minded activities rank so low that you seldom if ever get around to doing them by day's end. No shame in admitting that truth. The majority of people feel this way, which explains why 36.6 percent of Americans are overweight and 26.5 percent are obese. What's more, statistics point to the same thing happening overseas. The entire globe needs to reach for a bigger belt to cinch up its expanding waistline.

The simplest answer is that you're better off taking whatever time you need to get in that workout. A good workout can be wrapped in 45 minutes to an hour, the length of the typical Formula 50 workout. If you're like many people, you blow that much time messing around on Twitter or Facebook.

Eating healthfully takes time, but so does eating poorly. The better you plan, the less time healthy eating will consume. In fact, eating well can be made, if not faster than fast food, more efficiently. For example, you could prepare a week's worth of meals on a Sunday night; in contrast, you need to hit the drive-through every time you want a meal. Try saving *that* stuff in the fridge, and prepare to watch a chemistry experiment unfold in reverse. And the worst of that junk doesn't even decompose for weeks, a dead giveaway that you're eating nothing but chemicals and preservatives.

But working out is not a zero sum game, where you take time from something else, devote it to fitness instead, and have it be a wash. Being fit makes you more efficient in the other aspects of your life. Suddenly, you feel more energized when you wake up in the morning, and this natural buzz stays with you throughout the day. No longer do you slump after lunch or need a nap after work, which, together, probably drains more time than your workout did.

This is what's called a virtuous cycle, in which good things are feeding back on and amplifying each other. You may be more familiar with a vicious cycle, where the negatives in your life amount to a giant echo chamber of defeat and harmful influences.

Sound eating feeds back into the workouts, which in turn makes you crave healthy foods, which you know will fuel your body, because it's telling you just that.

## 2. I tried it before, and it didn't work. Why should I try again?

Many, many people who start on workout plans don't complete them. There are many, many reasons for this, and sometimes it's the plan's fault. It might just be a bad system or approach, perhaps designed by someone unqualified to do so. It probably wouldn't work for anybody. Or it may have been a decent or even good plan, only prescribed for the wrong person or at the wrong time. Maybe the subject loved outdoor workouts, but the program was a gym based hardcore bodybuilding workout. Wrong program, wrong person, wrong result. A good workout has to be one that encourages the person to work out. If the workout doesn't get someone ready and psyched for the next workout, the program failed, even if it looked great on paper.

Both of these scenarios are a shame because these people were ready to transform. Now that they've given it their best, only to fail, they'll be far less likely to try again in the future. In that sense, it's doubly unfortunate. The effects of failure may persist for much longer than this single attempt.

More often, the blame rests with those who stopped. The program was well tailored for their situation, and it would have worked, but they didn't stick with it. Sometimes it's just that simple: They weren't sufficiently motivated to get it done. It doesn't mean they're bad people, or that they'll always fail, but in this one instance, they dropped the ball. It happens to the best of us.

Here's the thing. The right fitness plan followed diligently works almost every time, barring one X factor—an injury. It's uncanny, really, but fitness done right is money in the bank when it comes to producing results. The human body responds predictably to the right fuel and exercise. The degree and speed of change may vary, but change happens, just like it does when you're unintentionally upsizing. If you sit on the sofa all day eating Cheetos, most of you will gain excess pounds. The body is doing what it does.

I love that about fitness: You can't write a check for it. Even the Money Team can't buy this one. You have to earn it. A guy living in the desert who works hard can produce better gains than someone paying a trainer $200 an hour in Beverly Hills. It's about heart and dedication.

### 3. I don't have good genetics. I'm not going to look like a fitness model anyway.

I hear this a lot, and it always makes me scratch my head. True, we're all different, and some people are blessed with more natural advantages than others. I might be more genetically inclined to put on muscle; you might be programmed to set fat ablaze like a five-alarm fire. As we both work out, our genetic endowment will guide us in that direction. But our workouts, meal plans, and environment will also help dictate our results over time.

This isn't like football or basketball, where your team is trying to beat their team. It's not like Floyd staring down his opponent. In fitness, the competition pits you against you. You want to become the best version of yourself that you possibly can. It may not be the sort of perfection seen on magazine covers, but do you care? That exposure is fleeting and doesn't pay much money anyway, according to my coauthor, a guy who has worked for the top magazines. I think you'll be surprised at how good you can be. You may not even recognize the man or woman in the mirror once you finish Formula 50. This is You 2.0, new and improved.

### 4. I don't live near a gym, and I couldn't afford one even if I did.

There are people for whom this is a problem, no doubt. But let me break this down. First, while my Formula 50 is a gym-based program, even those without access to a gym can still do the cardio and many of the resistance training exercises, or at least copycat-type moves. If you can't do a bench press, a push-up can do the trick. If you don't have dumbbells, you can still do a lunge. Nature is really one giant gym as well. Unless your neighborhood is too tough, anyone can go outside and bust out a good workout.

Most people, however, can find a gym near enough to attend. Try finding one that's on the way to work, so that you can grab a workout before or after work, or during your lunch break. Look around to find one that feels comfortable. If you're intimidated, you won't attend no matter what. If you're low-key and chill, you may not want to hear plates crashing on the floor around you and people screaming at the top of their lungs. Or maybe you do. But at least you'll know that and choose accordingly. Of course, price will be a big consideration for many of you. Don't be afraid to negotiate. I'm a hustler and like to cut the best deal I can get. That doesn't change no matter how much money I have sitting in the bank.

### 5. Every time I talk about working out and losing weight, my family members—who are also overweight and out of shape—ridicule me for the idea.

One of the crazier aspects of fitness is how the effort you make to better yourself can be met with a lack of support or even resentment. Shouldn't it be the opposite? This reminds me of what it's like to try and break out of the hood, with people wanting to hold you back because they don't have what it takes to leave. Your success reminds them, reinforces for them, that they can't make it. Rather than follow your lead, they would rather pull you back to them—even if doing so prevents you from enjoying all the benefits of working out: more self-esteem, more energy, better health, and so forth.

They're wrong and you're right. Nobody who truly cares for you should begrudge you trying to get into great shape. If you need to explain to them what you're doing and why you're doing it, fine; but once you've done that, keep going. Eventually, they'll come around, and if they don't, that's their problem. I guarantee you that for every family member or close friend who resents your efforts, maybe even tries to discourage you, twenty more will encourage you. The majority rules in this case.

### 6. I'm so damn out of shape that I'll never be able to lose this weight.

Even if you're not overweight, mustering the energy and effort to start working out can seem like a challenge. The longer you go without training, the harder "the comeback" seems. It becomes even more daunting when you add pounds. Suddenly, you realize it's going to take work, real work, just to return to where you started. Now imagine that someone has gained more than a little extra weight, maybe a few hundred pounds' worth. Not only is the psychological barrier daunting but now your overweight body is its own worst enemy. The one tool needed to fix you is itself damaged or broken. *God, how did I ever let myself get so out of shape*, you might say to yourself . . .

No matter how far you've fallen from being fit, you can still get back in the game. The human body is amazing at adaptation. That's why we're all still here. It responds fast when you start exercising and eating properly. You can shape up far more quickly than you fell out of shape. Been slacking for 10 years? In 1 year, one-tenth the time, you can get into great shape again. I'm not recommending a 10-year backslide. The internal damage from obesity doesn't go away as easily as a gut or flabby arms. But if you're in a hole, or you feel like you are, you can dig your way out of it. It's not too late.

Taking that first step can be hard. However, once you fight through that initial resistance of mind and body, fitness becomes easier. Just as your body changes quickly, so can your mind. The bad habits that made you fall out of shape might have formed over years, if not decades. But in a matter of weeks, if you stay the course, new patterns of positive behavior can replace the old negative ways. People who never changed their ways were so close. I think of someone lost in the forest, needing to walk only half a mile to find food and shelter, but who ended up dying from starvation and exposure. He had no idea how close he was to rescuing himself. Neither do many of you.

### 7. I don't know what to do in the gym. It seems intimidating to me.

Fear can affect your perception, making a threat seem bigger than it really is. In one study, participants with a fear of spiders were asked to undergo live encounters with tarantulas and, afterward, to estimate their size. The more afraid a participant said they were, the larger their estimate. A lot of it was all in their head.

Formula 50 will cut your gym fears down to size. I've been working out for years, and I enlisted the help of leading exercise experts in putting together this program. Still, you might feel uncertainty about starting any program, especially if you've never trained before. It's understandable. You're wearing unfamiliar clothes you're not used to wearing. People you're not used to seeing surround you. You're doing physical movements that may seem unfamiliar to you. It's hard to feel at home when it feels like all eyes are on you, just waiting for you to do something stupid and silly.

No one's watching you, at least not for very long. See those mirrors all over the gym? That's what people are looking at for the most part—their reflection. Some are checking their form, some are narcissistic, and some have nowhere else to look in between sets. Sorry to break it to you, BUT THEY DON'T CARE ABOUT YOU! In the gym, it's all me-me-me. Use that to your advantage. Relax.

Even if they WERE looking at you, they know where you're at. I can personally guarantee, with the same assurance of death and taxes, that every single person in the gym had their first day or session. They know the drill. And they don't care.

With each new workout, you'll feel more comfortable and self-assured. You'll begin to understand gym customs. You'll walk in between someone doing curls and the mirror, the guy or girl will shoot you a look, and you'll know not to do that again. That's how we become socialized in any field of endeavor. Your confidence will leap as you begin seeing results. Eventually, you'll be one of the veterans, and somebody will walk in front of you by mistake. Always remember, you were in their place once.

## 8. I'm not overweight, so I'm already in shape without training or adhering to a healthy eating plan.

Not so fast. Ever heard the term skinny fat? That refers to someone who, while from all appearances is thin, is actually a fat person on the inside, where it counts. Metabolically obese is the more technical term. This individual will have the same problems a fat dude or heavyset girl is saddled with: high triglycerides, high blood pressure, bum cholesterol scores, high blood sugar or even diabetes, and related problems. If you put this person on a treadmill, he or she would be huffing and puffing just as prematurely as the bigs would.

Fitness is about more than body weight, and being normal weight but inactive can bring a false sense of security. *Oh, I can eat this*, you think. *It doesn't make me gain weight, so what's the big deal anyway?* Well, the big deal is the hardening of your arteries and the heart attack to come as a result. The heavyset person will be urged to lose weight by everyone from friends and family to their doctor, but you won't be. No one will think to say anything to you.

## 9. I don't want to be one of those people carrying Tupperware full of stinky fish into meetings at work. Ugh.

This sounds like a joke, but it hits on a key point: the feeling that working out and all that goes with it isn't cool. Instead of stylin', suddenly you're carrying around a gym bag, and having to change and shower in the middle of the day, and packing meals in little plastic containers filled with boring food shoved into a cooler, which then has to be lugged to and from work. How can you be the lion in the room with a little container of chicken and broccoli sitting before you? The worst stereotype is the bodybuilder whose life is ruled by frequent feedings and several workouts a day, leaving little room for anything else. Anything but cool.

You can be fit and not do any of this. My meal plans are designed so that you eat three meals a day, plus a snack. No need to be Tupperware Boy or Girl. My nutrition guru, Layne Norton, PhD, has research showing that spreading your meals out doesn't really hasten fat burning, as has often been reported. So I have you follow a more traditional regimen, one that should fit easily within your lifestyle. Breakfast, lunch, dinner, snack. That's it. Probably how you're eating now, only now the foods will be much healthier and chosen with purpose.

But above and beyond all this, fitness is now cool. Taking care of oneself is attractive. Looking good is prized. People are smarter and hipper than ever. They understand you don't get fit in a vacuum, that it's the byproduct of a lifestyle that takes some work. They connect the dots when they see someone with a great body who leaves the office holding a gym bag, or drinking a protein shake instead of a Coke. Getting the flab off of your hips is now hip.

**10.** My garage is full of fitness equipment I picked up on HSN and QVC. All it's doing is collecting dust. That's proof that I can't do this!

It's not that fitness isn't for you; it's that you've been going about it all wrong. Fitness isn't about buying something on a home-shopping network and then expecting it to work miracles. Most of the apparatuses don't work as well as free weights, gym machines, and even body-weight moves for starters. Some of it's okay, some of it is junk, but none of it is the best way to work out. Fitness is a business, and some really smart marketing minds have figured out what buttons to push. They don't know what makes people fit, but they sure know what makes people whip out their credit cards to pay for a quick fix.

This doesn't mean you can't get in shape; it just means you need to go about it the right way this time. I know the term sounds more New Age than hip-hop, but what you need is a holistic approach that trains your muscles, your cardiovascular system, and your flexibility with many different exercises in many different ways, coupled with sound nutritional practices. That works. Once you realize that, you can easily do this exercise: Lift those apparatuses off the garage floor and dump them in the trash. You don't need that stuff anymore.

## Patience Makes Perfect

In the hip-hop world people often have great interest in things they shouldn't. I'll ride through the roughest neighborhoods in South Jamaica and Brooklyn, and I'll see people on the corners in Gucci, Louis Vuitton, and Nikes—but the $200 Nikes, because when we look good, we feel good. Wear that clothing and it gives you instant gratification, temporary confidence, a quick fix. Credibility.

There are better ways to achieve those feelings, ways that make them last, like working out and sculpting your body. We all yearn for immediate results, but unlike buying a new pair of kicks, getting into shape is a process. I don't go into the studio and leave the next day with a masterpiece bangin' in my headphones. Likewise, if you decide to learn how to dance because your wedding is 2 weeks away, you probably harbor no illusions of dancing like Chris Brown at that point. If you decide to pick up tennis because of a business-related match next month, you probably don't expect to be Wimbledon caliber by that point in time.

Don't live in a fantasy world. Be realistic. You have to put in the time. Dedication is a must. You have to allow your body to respond to the new demands you're placing on it. Meaningful achievements take time, and becoming fit is no exception. You'll need that patience for the long haul, because it's harder to keep up the rate of improvement over time. Someone who is 100 pounds overweight can look like a different human being after a few months of weight loss, whereas a fitness fanatic will make less dramatic improvements, having started from a higher level. The rate of progress tends to level off, but it levels off with you being fitter and healthier than you were before. That's winning.

It's different from the sort of plateau-bound inertia or even regression that occurs when you don't change up your workouts. You'll notice that Formula 50 changes things up all the time. The changes might be subtle, like your rest in between sets decreasing from 45 seconds to 30. But those are the kind of changes that keep your body adapting (good) rather than stagnating (bad).

Part of being patient is not being so hard on yourself. Learn how to relax and just say, "It's cool." We're not perfect. We all make mistakes. But hard work is rewarded in the end. I have had times in my life when I was angry, especially with some of the things I dealt with as a kid. Growing up without a father, losing my mother at age 8, dealing crack, getting shot—none of it was easy. Training has helped me be better with people and better with myself. Being patient and not judging myself so harshly. If you judge yourself harshly, you want to pick at other people too. That's why I feel like people bully other people—because it makes them feel better about themselves. *Maybe* I'm *not so great, but look at her. I don't do that.*

People think that because I'm nicknamed The Machine that anything having to do with fitness should come easy for me. As a result, they might think I would be very hard on people who are overweight. While there is a place for tough love, I'm more into results-driven motivation. I don't judge others based on body weight; those out-of-shape individuals may be happier than me for all I know. I just know how much better they'd feel in their own skin if they ditched that excess weight.

You'll hear news reports all the time about some new gene that may be responsible for making more than half of America fat. People with this gene may be more likely to become obese, but genetics only loads the gun. The lifestyle choices you make are what pull the trigger. We've become six times more obese in the last 50 years, but our genetics certainly haven't changed that dramatically in one or two generations. Something more is at work.

Even our pets are in the midst of an obesity epidemic! Their genetics didn't change all of a sudden either. It's just that all of these animals had survived throughout history by being thrifty with calories, and now that calories are so prevalent, many of those same species are becoming overweight. First it was our adults who became obese. Then it was our children who became obese. Now it's our pets that are getting fat. That's crazy, man.

We live in a society where people are always looking to pass the buck. "Oh, don't worry, it's not your fault. It's your DNA's fault or McDonald's fault or somebody else's fault." People know McDonald's food isn't healthy for them, by and large, but they eat there anyway. You make the decisions.

# 4

# Why MRT Is So Smart

I

F FAILURE IS ONE OF YOUR FEARS, ARE YOU READY TO FACE IT head-on? If it's your first attempt, I know it's not easy stepping through that door for the first time. For this not to be your first attempt poses its own set of challenges. You need to understand why it's going to work this time, when it didn't work before.

The scene you encounter inside might be sedate and non-threatening, but it could just as easily be as intense as one of my concerts, what with all the grinding, clanging, and yelling going on. If you think female tennis players grunt loudly during their matches, wait till you hear serious weight trainers getting after it in the gym.

One thing you'll notice is that in your typical gym, the vast majority of the square footage is occupied by long rows of fancy machines. The barbells and dumbbells, or free weights, are usually racked up in the back, with a little space cleared out for actually using them. But the weights themselves probably take up less space than the juice bar does.

Don't let the percentages fool you. They may take up the least amount of space, but free weights produce the biggest and best results. When it comes to fitness, technology, in the form of machines, is not the be-all and end-all. Your biggest foe with free weights is gravity, and it never gives an inch, doesn't care how tired you are that day, doesn't want to hear about what a jerk your boss is.

Think about doing a leg extension versus doing a squat. If you can't finish the last rep of a leg extension, you gently lower the pad back down and pull yourself from out of the machine. If the same thing happens on a squat, *Damn—What do I do now?* You need true strength to handle that load, or else. There may be a higher risk with free weights, but you'll receive the best instruction there is in this book. And the rewards are so much higher than they are with machines.

Machines are comfy, no doubt. They also seem simple in that they hit one muscle at a time. For legs, there's the leg machine. For chest, there's the chest machine. And so on, all aligned down the row. The problem comes when you leave the gym. Life doesn't happen one muscle group at a time. You don't find yourself in that same position, needing to curl your biceps, 4 hours later. Instead, you need to reach down and grab your kid, who tries to scramble when he's a few inches off the ground. Every muscle in your body tenses, your joints are hit with unexpected forces, your spine turns unnaturally, and you find yourself off balance.

Your body has never experienced this before. But it knows how to do a machine curl. Remind yourself of that as you and your kid hit the deck.

The bigger free-weight exercises accustom your body to moving in space, with a variety of joint and muscles synchronized and nothing to brace you. This is called compound training, and it leads to much better results than tons of machine moves, both in terms of how you look and how you perform out in the real world.

The Formula 50 workout programs are built around compound moves, and not by accident: Joe Dowdell and I know they produce the sort of internal body responses capable of generating a 50-percent improvement over the 6 weeks on the beginner's plan, as well as even more dramatic gains if you continue on with the advanced program. That's not to say you'll find no machine moves in the programs. We use them selectively, and with a specific goal in mind anytime we do. However, they are exceptions to this rule: Free weights and body-weight moves rule on Formula 50.

It's your prerogative to train this way or not. I'm just telling you what produces the best results.

## So Where Did All That Fat Come from in the First Place?

I'm guessing many of you picked up this book because you're trying to ditch some weight. The first thing to realize is that weight gain and weight loss doesn't produce the neat "calories in, calories out" math you often see in magazines or hear on TV. Take an obese person who has been living on Big Macs and large Cokes for 20 years. Their excess baggage is what remains after subtracting what they should weigh from their current fat-inflated weight. Were you to divide that excess-baggage number by the total number of days in question, you might calculate that they had to consume, say, 10 calories a day extra over the years to accumulate all that fat.

Now put someone on a diet that reduces their consumption by 10 calories a day. Guess what? You wouldn't see any difference. That reduction alone would be a meaningless change, even if it were extended indefinitely. How is that possible? Shouldn't the same thing work in reverse?

When it comes to the foods we eat, our bodies aren't simple calorie counters, and our body weight isn't the difference between calories in and calories out, even though we've been told that for decades. Take carbohydrates and protein. One gram of each contains 4 calories. However, for every 100 grams of carbs consumed, the body "nets" only 93. In contrast, for every 100 grams of protein consumed, only 70 make the cut. The body spends far more energy digesting protein than carbs. Which means too much happens between the "in" and the "out" parts for that equation to be accurate.

Exercise is similar in certain respects. People will say, "Okay, if I want to lose weight, I'll walk a mile to burn 100 calories. If I walk 5 miles, I'll burn 500 calories. So, I'll lose a pound a week." Off they go on their power walks, confident that their weight-loss calculations will lead to weight loss and transformation.

They might lose 1 pound that first week. Maybe they'll lose another the next week. Then the body realizes something's changing, and it swings back toward *homeostasis*— internal stability in the face of opposing forces, kind of like the peacemaker in a rap war. The body does so by slowing its metabolic rate. It's saying, *Hold up yo. If you're going to expend energy by walking around all the time, I'm going to expend less energy when you're sleeping and sitting. Because we might need it later.*

No wonder you sometimes see even fitness people doing 2 hours of cardio a day with little or no weight loss to show for it. Their metabolic rate has become glacial. So the net result is a big FAT zero. Talk about exercise in futility.

Weight training and high-intensity intervals are just about the only kinds of exercise that don't slow your metabolic rate. They increase it. That's why these forms of exercise are crucial for maintaining—not just achieving—a healthy body weight. Formula 50 uses these techniques because they burn fat and increase muscle. Your sets will be so intense that they'll exhaust your oxygen and strengthen your heart faster and more efficiently than endless treadmill walking.

I'm not going to have you do just any kind of weight training, however. Your lifting sessions, like your cardio, will be highly metabolic in nature. That's the source of the name metabolic resistance training, or MRT. It's the most sophisticated approach to changing body composition through training, ripped straight from America's exercise science labs.

## Make Science Your Ally in Fat Loss

There was a time, long before my "In Da Club" video, when "lab" with "exercise" would never have been uttered in the same sentence. So a lot of sketchy theories were hatched in basements and then spouted off in gyms, even if they were total BS. One guy might have preached that 50 sets on the bench press done four times a week is the key to building big pectorals, when in truth, it will push you into a state of overtraining and slow your progress. Another guy might have been convinced that 2 hours of daily cardio was the key to effective fat loss. More BS, but no one really knew better.

Much of this info was "bro-science"—nonsense with no rhyme or reason. Dudes at the gym throwing around puny weight and using big words, but clueless.

Researchers have been catching up with a vengeance since around 1990. The last decade in particular has seen an outpouring of research into the metabolic aspects of exercise. In fact, exercise scientists have learned more in the past 10 years alone than they did in the prior 100. MRT is now gaining favor thanks to a lot of new, cutting-edge research. Those in the field now have a much better sense of what works and what doesn't.

The closest thing you may have experienced to MRT is circuit training, where you moved from one machine to the next, maybe 10 in all, to complete a circuit. It's been around for a while, and people have mostly done it for efficiency's sake rather than as a fat-burning strategy. But it turned out that this style of training was more aerobic than traditional weight training had been. It also could lead to greater body fat reduction. All well and good, but your parents' circuit training was really only a blueprint for Formula 50's version of MRT.

Back then, not much attention was paid to manipulating workout intensity or developing functional strength and agility. You moved robotically from machine to machine and then hit the showers. Still, it was an attempt to bring an aerobic component to weight training, and in that sense, it was a precursor of sorts to this program—but only in the sense that a Model T predated the Ferrari. Big difference.

Despite circuit training's obvious appeal for the time crunched, stressed-out masses, most people still thought of cardio as one thing, weights as another thing, and flexibility training as the third pillar of a "fitness triad." More advanced forms of MRT, like those in Formula 50, break the mold. An exercise physiologist I've come to know and respect, Brad Schoenfeld, MSC, master of science in exercise science, CSCS, lecturer in exercise science at Lehman College, explains it this way: "Anaerobic training, resistance training, and aerobic training consist on a continuum. They're different in terms of the energy pathways that are 'up-regulated,' but the lines between them begin to blur if you look at the research."

The blurring isn't just between resistance training and cardio, but between resistance training and flexibility training. Brad's rollin' here, so I'll let him continue: "The old thought that resistance training would make you muscle bound and less flexible has also gone by the wayside. There is now quite a bit of research showing that resistance training actually improves flexibility." Those who resistance train are more flexible than those who don't as a result.

That myth about muscle-bound bodybuilders being inflexible developed because a true hardcore bodybuilder, the 'roid beast rocking 25-inch guns, simply has so much muscle that it gets in the way of his ability to move through a range of motion. The muscles themselves aren't any less flexible, however.

## The Balanced Way to Build Your Body

To bring elements of your cardio training into your weight workouts, it helps to understand what's happening inside your body while you exercise. Exercise requires energy, and the body contains different energy pathways. Some pathways are anabolic, meaning they lead to muscle growth. The word *anabolic* has a negative connotation because it's often used to modify the word *steroid*, but other processes can be anabolic. Lifting weights is anabolic. Drinking a protein shake is anabolic. A good night's sleep is anabolic. And, yes, certain "pharmaceuticals," taken illegally, are also anabolic. But that's not what I'm talking about here.

The body also has pathways that are catabolic, which is the opposite of anabolic. During a catabolic process, tissue is broken down rather than built up. You may be thinking, *Man, why would I want to do that?* Well, to give you one example, you have to be catabolic to break down fat.

It's hard to be anabolic and catabolic at the same time, but the Formula 50 program seeks to do just that. You may not build muscle as fast as you would on a purely muscle-building program—but you will build muscle. You may not burn fat quite as fast as you would on a purely fat-burning program—but you will burn fat. What's more, your conditioning will improve more than either of those approaches would allow. Finally, your body composition will shift to promote continuous fat burning for a long time.

Trade-offs come with the territory. It's hard to develop a ton of size with MRT, especially because the diet portion is fairly low in carbs. This is not a program for turning yourself into a mass monster. But you will add lean tissue to your frame. My coauthor gained 10 pounds of muscle during 6 weeks on the program.

How about strength? With MRT, the rest periods are too short to allow you to trigger higher-threshold motor units, which must be tapped into to develop dramatically higher strength as measured by the one-rep maximum. But for everyday living and fitness, strength endurance is what you really want to improve. This is your strength staying power, your stamina when push comes to shove and you need to hold something for an extended period of time. To me, that's real strength, not the strength that's all show and no go.

Circuit training strikes a great balance between maintaining muscle and shedding body fat. One of the things that circuit training and other MRT techniques allow is a greater post-exercise effect than just weight training or just cardio alone. Steady state cardio, in fact, produces very little post-workout fat burning.

In contrast, the Formula 50 workouts—especially if you're doing them as intensely as you should—can keep the fat burning strong for 48 or even 72 hours afterward. Instead of doing the sort of circuit training where you try to move with no rest, you're going to maybe take 60 seconds or fewer. I also like to pair muscle groups so the muscle itself is allowed some rest. So you would do a shoulder press (a push) and then a lat pull-down (a pull). Or a chest press followed by a row. That way you're not taxing the same muscle; you're allowing it a little bit of rest even while you're still training.

MRT also primes your ability to increase lactate threshold. This is your body's ability to clear lactic acid from muscle tissue. Lactic acid results in fatigue and creates "the burn." MRT conditions your body to have a higher lactate set point, which will increase your ability to crank out reps later, during times when you're not training this way. Once your body learns to clear lactate more readily, instead of getting 10 reps with a certain weight, you may get 11 or 12. This should lead to more muscle growth. So not only is this training style going to work great while you're on the Formula 50 program, it will also pay dividends long afterward, whether you're advanced, intermediate, or starting out.

What's more, that original selling point for circuit training—efficiency—still holds true for the Formula 50 style of MRT. General fitness enthusiasts are often pressed for time, and it can get nuts when you're working all day and then coming home to deal with kids. None of those people has 2 hours to spend in the gym. They want a big bang for their buck, and those concerned about building muscle and burning fat receive a nice mixture.

MRT is also nearly unrivaled when it comes to overall conditioning. Your lung capacity and heart health will both improve quickly on Formula 50. So this is the perfect compromise solution for someone who wants general fitness, toned muscle, and less fat. Train smart and you can have it all.

## The Language of Lifting

- Your "workout" is composed of the exercises you will do that day.
- An "exercise" is the type of movement you use to lift the weight. Examples: bench press, squat, sit-up, etc. An exercise is composed of "repetitions" and "sets."
- A "repetition" is one complete lift, from starting position (extension) to maximum contraction, and back to starting position (extension).
- A "set" is a group of nonstop repetitions (i.e., "two sets of 10 repetitions" means 10 nonstop repetitions, rest, and another 10 nonstop repetitions).
- A "body part" (muscle group) is one of the following: chest, shoulders, back, biceps, triceps, legs, or abdominals.

During the advanced phase of Formula 50, you'll engage in combo training, which is a little different from super setting and circuit training, in that you're doing bursts of aerobic activity in between sets. This is the most challenging style of MRT on the planet, depending on how it's done. What I really like about it—besides its effectiveness—is how efficient it becomes to do high-intensity aerobic type work in between your lifts. When you're training like this, you really don't need straightforward aerobic training. You're doing jumping jacks, squat thrusts, some heavy-duty calisthenics, even high-stepping in between your sets. This all has a huge metabolic effect—which is exactly what we're after.

# 5

# Nearly Everything You Know About Dieting Is Wrong

**W**HAT YOU EAT OR DON'T EAT LARGELY DETERmines whether you gain body fat, lose body fat, or hold steady. You can exercise most days, but if those workouts are bookended by burgers and chocolate shakes, chances are you're not going to look anything near the guy or girl on the cover of a fitness magazine.

Think of the best physical condition you've ever experienced. We're going to top it. But it won't happen by accident; I need you to nourish your body a certain way. Am I putting you on a diet? The wording matters much less than the meaning does. If it *is* a diet, it's a diet in the original Greek sense of the term—a style of life, a way of being. People often fail at "dieting" because they treat it as a side activity rather than making healthy eating part of their lifestyle. As for people who are in shape, well, they seldom say they're eating something *because they're on a diet.* They just eat that way every day.

Too often, people gear up to diet and then choose a plan as repetitive and boring as some terrible beat stuck in your head. These crash diets typically have one goal, and that's weight loss. But the plans are shortsighted, diverting attention from what really matters: the shift in body composition that comes from losing fat and gaining muscle. So dieters drag themselves along in misery, as if walking a prison yard for a long line of past dietary indiscretions. The complaints will be constant, to the point where you don't want to be near those people. They're depriving themselves, and they want you and the rest of the world to know it. Misery loves company.

Often, these people will actually drop some weight during the first weeks of their diet. So far, so good, right? Only there's usually a problem lurking: They're not making dietary changes a lasting part of their lifestyle. They're not enjoying what they're eating; they're enduring it. But having lost at least some weight, they'll pat themselves on the back for a job well done. Then they ditch the diet and go back to their old menu.

It's not a job, and it wasn't well done. In a cruel twist, those folks are doomed to gain back that weight and more! See, when someone diets, 60 percent of what they lose typically is fat tissue, while the other 40 percent is lean tissue, or muscle. So if this hypothetical person were to lose 10 pounds, for example, 6 would be fat pounds and 4 would be muscle pounds. Unfortunately, when the person reverts to the old ways of eating, the weight comes back. Only what comes back is almost exclusively fat. So they're worse off than when they started. Anyone who's ever gone on a deprivation diet likely has experienced this unpleasant boomerang effect.

No wonder people view dieting as such a monumental struggle.

Many dieters fail to realize just how important lean muscle is for long-term fat burning. If you leave this book with one concept fixed in your mind, this should be it: Muscle burns fat. A lot of your insulin sensitivity and other fat-burning tools are tied directly to your body's total reserves of lean tissue. So as your body composition (the ratio of muscle to fat) changes, you'll burn more calories as a result. No matter what you're doing, even if you're sleeping, you're burning more calories than you were before. It all adds up.

You can't blame the people promoting these bum diets. Well, you could, but it wouldn't matter. It is what it is. The individuals hustling these plans tend to focus on the dieter achieving some measurable reduction in pounds during the first 2 weeks. They want you to feel like something good is happening. *Wow, look! The scale says I'm losing weight! Yay!* Yet once those dieters revert to their former eating patterns, they gain back all that weight and more. Now they're worse off than they were before. Better they had not dieted at all. At least they wouldn't have surrendered their precious fat-burning muscle tissue.

What's sad is that most of these people who are struggling with their weight already have been on this diet merry-go-round. They're more concerned with looking good than feeling good. Why are they "dieting" in the first place? Maybe they look in the mirror, see extra "pudge" that wasn't there during their teen years, and decide to do something about it. But they don't change their lifestyle. They diet, lose some pounds, and then regain the weight.

They go through cycles of trying different diets, one after the other, losing less weight each time, gaining back even more weight each time. They reach a point where they start a new diet, like they have many times before, and yet can't lose ANY weight. Which sounds crazy, right? How does dieting lead dieters down a path to a place where they become prisoners of their metabolism, trapped in their own overweight bodies?

Depriving yourself, and losing some of that lean tissue each time you do, impairs your long-term fat-burning ability. You've bumped down your metabolism so many times that your body can no longer respond even to a deprivation diet. That's when the unwanted pounds begin piling up. You may have heard about or even seen people who spend 2 hours a day on the treadmill, eat 1,000 calories a day, and yet can't lose any weight. They didn't do it the right way. They made their sole focus weight loss, rather than learning how to lose body fat and support muscle growth.

I'm not just talking about overweight truck drivers and accountants either. Take fitness competitors, some of the most disciplined dieters and exercisers on earth. Many of them go through highly restrictive stretches of eating when preparing for a contest, only to binge as soon as they shed their bikini. When they repeat this cycle a few different times, they also start struggling to lose weight. They can't shed pounds, because they've repeatedly beaten down their metabolism. They *look* like they're in shape, but their metabolism is sputtering.

Weight loss starts with a lifestyle change. Think marathon, not sprint. Of course losing body fat involves some measure of calorie restriction. But if you start a diet that limits you to eating only a certain type of protein source, or only fruit, or only a certain *type* of fruit, even—remember the grapefruit diet?—it usually won't be maintained. Life interferes. Christmas, anniversaries, business dinners, and other social obligations require flexibility. Who wants to be the stick-in-the-mud all the time? If you go over to Grandma's house, and she's cooked you a big pot of spaghetti, what are you going to say? "I'm sorry, Grandma, but I can't eat that because I'm dieting"? Most people won't understand that. There has to be enough flexibility for you to enjoy non-diet foods with portion control.

What if I told you that you could eat normally at those events and make much more progress than you've been making to date? That you'll finally achieve weight loss that can be maintained lifelong? That's a promise from me to you, right here and now: Follow the Formula 50 plan, and when holidays roll around, you can do what you want. The results will still amaze you because you'll be acing the program on the other days.

## Fat, Meet Your Worst Nightmare: Muscle

Now that I've explained why most diets fail, let me explain why the Formula 50 meal plan works. You have to start by changing how you view your body and nutrition. Instead of thinking about losing weight, start thinking about gaining muscle. Muscle, you see, is the true fat fighter.

If I walk up to the average woman and say, "You could use another 10 pounds of muscle," she'll probably say, "Well, I don't want to get too bulky." Listen: Muscle looks good! The folks in the magazines don't end up looking that way by accident. That is a very purposeful, focused, often decade-long effort to become as muscular as possible. You're looking at the end result of a Commitment, capital c.

Most people benefit from adding a few muscle pounds. The amount of muscle you have is closely tied to not only how long you live but also how healthfully you live. As it turns out, muscle does all sorts of dope things. Muscle sends out and receives hormone signals, a sort of "cross talk" between muscle tissue and the brain.

Dr. Norton makes a good point. Why not treat muscle with some respect? If you went to the doctor and learned your liver was unhealthy, the doctor delivering the news would be pretty concerned, right? But if you went to your doctor and said, "Yo, doc, I think my muscle is pretty unhealthy," you would probably be laughed out the door. Or the doc would say, "Whatever. It's just muscle. You don't want to look too big anyway."

So what about people carrying a lot of muscle? Are they a heart attack waiting to happen, as some would suggest, or are they healthier than the average person? Let's take the extreme case of the power lifter, someone whom most people would think is not only big but also overweight. Most of those guys carry extra weight on purpose. They know the added bulk will help them lift heavy objects in strength events. But those same guys can lose body fat fast when needed. Underneath that extra layer of padding, those strong dudes have big, metabolically active muscles, allowing them to gear up on cue for fat loss.

That muscle gives them the benefit of using calories in ways that are beneficial rather than harmful. I'll illustrate this using a construction analogy.

Let's say that at a certain point the road leading to your office forks into a Y. The roads merge back into one lane a few miles later. You can go left, or you can go right, but regardless, you'll end up at the same place.

Now let's say a construction crew whips out the orange signs and walkie-talkies and starts blocking off the lane of traffic that veers to the left. Anyone who's not consciously trying to kill time will now go to the right because no obstruction looms. That's a form of *partitioning*. Traffic is being partitioned based on the actions taken by the road crew.

Like those drivers, nutrients in the body also choose between two paths: the muscle path and the fat path. When you work out, you make muscle tissue active, which in turn makes the muscle path the chosen one. There are no walkie-talkies, but your body commands nutrients, "Go this way." At the same time, muscle tells fat, "Fuhgeddaboudit—you're not getting these nutrients. We demand them." When you work out—especially with weights or just your own body versus gravity—muscle becomes greedy, and it starts bullying around fat and hogging all the calories. The benefit is twofold: It's not just that you're building muscle; it's that those calories that could have ended up as fat now go elsewhere.

There's an alternative scenario that plays out across the land every day. If you're sitting around on the sofa, your muscles have no need for greed. How much energy does it take to click the remote and go grab a soft drink or beer? If you're lounging, it doesn't take much fuel to satisfy muscle's needs. This allows fat cells to become greedy. And fat cells have an unlimited capacity to absorb excess calories.

## Can Eating Burn Calories? It's *Not* a Trick Question!

Another advantage of protein is the calories you burn digesting it, through what's called the thermic effect of food. Simply put, we all spend a certain amount of energy extracting energy from the foods we eat, whether it's a truck driver with his Whopper with cheese or a supermodel and her celery stick. How much energy your body needs to invest varies based on the type of food being consumed. Protein turns out to have a higher thermic effect than carbs and fat do. The difference isn't marginal, either. It's more like five- or sixfold higher.

No matter what you eat, your body always extracts more energy than it invests through digestion; the "net" is always a positive number. Yet because protein takes more energy to digest than other macros require, eating it burns more calories than dining on the other two sources does. Protein is "energetically expensive," because it activates muscle metabolism. It flicks the switch at a cellular level.

If muscle is so great at burning fat, and protein is so great at building muscle, how much should you consume to maximize these effects? You have to reach a certain threshold of protein intake before you start reaping its full benefits. If you take in, say, 5 grams' worth, I'm sorry to say, it won't do much—even if the protein comes from a high-quality source. You're just not getting enough protein to activate that growth signal or switch.

According to research relayed to me by Dr. Norton, for smaller people, often women, it appears that if your meal includes 20 grams of protein, there's a good chance you're going to surpass that threshold. If you're a little bit larger in size—talking mostly guys here—it probably takes more like 30 grams of high-quality protein in a meal to reach that threshold and flip the growth switch.

I'm generalizing based on Dr. Norton's information, and there are obviously differences among individuals, but these rules seem to apply for about 95 percent of people. As it turns out, blood levels of amino acids are not linear. Sounds technical, but let me break it down. Dr. Norton explains how people were fed 5, 10, 15, 20, or 30 grams of protein. Then their blood amino acids were tracked. At those lower protein intakes, there wasn't that much of a change. However, when subjects reached those

20- to 30-gram marks, all of a sudden, boom, it doubled. This coincided with a jump in protein synthesis.

Protein makes you much more insulin sensitive, meaning it reduces the amount of insulin needed to clear glucose from the bloodstream. Removing this glucose is important because too much glucose in your blood adds up to type 2 diabetes, a disease you want to avoid—and will avoid, if you follow my plan.

If you have only 10 or 15 pounds to lose, or you're looking to gain muscle, your target protein intake on my program is 0.8 to 1 gram per pound of body weight per day. If you weigh 200 pounds, consume upwards of 200 grams a day; if you weigh 155 pounds, consume upwards of 155 grams; and so on. Your protein should come from sources such as eggs and milk; lean meats such as lean beef, chicken, turkey, and fish; and whey protein powder. No deprivation here. All tasty stuff.

There are a few exceptions. Those of you who are very overweight should aim for 0.7 or 0.8 grams of protein per pound of body weight. In contrast, those of you who are really carb sensitive or even type 2 diabetic should add additional protein to replace some of your carbs.

You can also raise your carb threshold a bit by eating protein along with those starchy foods. In fact, adding muscle building protein gives you a higher tolerance for carbs. It does so by lowering the glycemic effect of those carbs. Protein again will activate muscle, making it more greedy, taking away some of those carbs so that fat doesn't get a crack at them. Protein does dietary damage control.

Research shows that eating protein at breakfast may reduce your food intake throughout the day. Consider a study by Dr. Norton's advisor. For 16 months, it was The Zone diet versus the food pyramid diet, so 40-30-30 (carb, protein, fat percentages) versus 55 percent carb, 15 percent protein, and 30 percent fat. They found that some members of the high protein group didn't even eat the amount of calories they were supposed to. They weren't hungry enough.

Think of your own experience. How many big bowls of cereal can you plow through if you're hungry? Two, three? How about bagels? You probably can sit down and eat two or three without thinking twice, good for 150 grams and 600 calories' worth of carbs. But as for protein . . . could you eat three chicken breasts in a sitting? Probably not. Chicken is weightier and more satisfying.

Unfortunately, most mainstream recommendations for protein, including the government's standard-issue recommendation, don't account for these factors. They give you your requirement, but your requirement may be very different from what's best for your health, especially when you're training hard—hence the higher protein recommendation in Formula 50. Trust me, this strategy will work wonders for you.

## The Carb Precipice—Watch Out!

On the other hand, our national dietary recommendations call for too many carbs, which is not the way to get lean. Carbs are sneaky; you have to keep an eye on 'em. Use them to your advantage, and they can become a great ally in your efforts to shape up. Abuse them, and they can sabotage the best-laid plans. Most of the overweight people in America have experienced this firsthand, whether they know it. Carbs, not fat, and definitely not protein, are often what make people fat.

The human body reacts to carbs with more variability than it does protein and fat. Due to these large differences in individual tolerance, carbs will be the most variable nutrient. Even more than with protein, the source of your carbs makes all the difference. A Ding Dong has a much different effect on your body than a sweet potato, even though both are carb foods.

Good carbs tend to be higher in fiber than bad carbs, which is what you want. These good carbs make you feel full, so you stop eating. On my plan, any carb that is at least 20 percent fiber is a quality source. So let's say you're strolling down the food store aisles and see two bread choices. One of 'em has 20 grams of carbs and 4 grams of fiber, and the other has 20 grams of carbs and 2 grams of fiber. Only the first one would be 50 Cent approved.

So what happens to carbs once they enter your body? Whenever you eat food, your gut tissues get first crack at it. So if your intestines need any energy, they take it. Then your liver takes what it needs. After that, your muscle tissue takes its share. Fat cells get the last shot.

Carbs have the same sort of patterns and thresholds as protein, but in reverse. Dr. Norton explained research that studied this phenomenon too. The question: What level of carb intake can you give someone to take care of the needs of gut tissues, the liver, and muscles without triggering fat storage? Again, I'm simplifying, but the threshold seems to be 30 to 40 grams of carbs. Go beyond that range in a meal, and those carbs will start turning into body fat. So you can see why fast food wrecks your diet and harms your health. Drink a Coke and eat fries and a burger bun, and you're easily way past that threshold. Heck, one 12-ounce can of Coke contains 39 grams of carbs, all simple sugars. Do it every day for a few years and your belly may need its own zip code.

When people say they're carb sensitive, what they're saying is they're insulin insensitive. There is an amount of insulin you need to clear a certain number of carbs, and below the cutoff points I mentioned—40 grams if you eat just carbs, 50 grams if you combine the carbs with protein—the amounts of insulin needed to clear the glucose is pretty small. However, beyond those levels, insulin secretion jumps. The more your insulin spikes to clear glucose over time, and the more times those insulin molecules hook up to the receptors on the cells, the less effective your body becomes at doing exactly that. It wears down this glucose-clearing ability; cells become insensitive to insulin.

The more insulin-insensitive the muscle becomes, the more insulin you need to dispose of the same amount of glucose. That insulin isn't just disposing of glucose; it's sending signals to your liver to make and store fat. Long-term increases in insulin secretion are inflammatory. They damage blood vessels. When you secrete a lot of insulin over a long period of time, that's bad. I'm not saying you can't ever have carbs. I'm not saying you can't ever have a bowl of cereal. But you're going to have to control your portion size.

## Start Strong: Breakfast Sets the Tone for Everything

What you eat at breakfast sets the tone for the rest of your day. The problem is that many of our very worst foods are clustered at this kick-off meal. Muffins, scones, pastries, doughnuts, home fries, sugary breakfast cereals—all are consumed for breakfast like clockwork by a wide swath of the population.

The numbers add up fast when you combine these foods. If you eat a bowl of cereal, 30 grams or so comes from half a cup, and nobody eats half a cup. Drink a glass of orange juice, maybe have a muffin—the grams start to pile up into the triple digits. People say, "Well, that cereal gives you some whole grains and fiber." Yeah, you may be getting 4 grams of fiber, but they aren't going to do much when measured against those 50 grams of carbs. To use one of Dr. Norton's expressions, that's like shooting a BB gun at a barge.

Perhaps convenience is to blame, but a lot of people either skip it or choose a big bowl of cereal or a bagel or toast. Honestly, if you are just eating carbs at breakfast, you're better off skipping it. Having only carbs is probably the worst thing you can do. The latest research suggests that having only carbs for breakfast sets you up for more snacking throughout the day.

So what have we done as a culture? Glorified carb-based breakfast foods and demonized eggs, which are an awesome breakfast food. Hello, diabetes epidemic. What's worse, oftentimes the carb sources people choose are also high fat. This creates a damaging mix of really high insulin, really high glucose, and really high fat. If you don't have any protein in there, you're basically opening a one-lane highway toward fat storage.

In the United States and other Western societies, most people consume about 65 percent of their protein at dinner. So if they're taking in 100 grams of protein in a day, 65 grams are coming at dinner. Which means they're having very little protein with breakfast and lunch, unfortunately. Dr. Norton's lab did a cool study to gauge the effects of how protein consumption was distributed throughout the day. Study subjects were fed the exact same protein intake, but one group received their protein in evenly distributed "doses" three times a day, while the other group got 70 percent at dinner, 15 percent at breakfast, and 15 percent at lunch.

People whose protein was dispersed equally had a little bit less fat, but they had significantly more muscle mass. As I've explained, that's what's most important for long-term body composition. It all goes back to hitting that protein threshold we talked about. What normally happens is that people don't hit that threshold at breakfast, they don't hit it at lunch, but then, finally, they hit it at dinner. The current recommendation of protein intake is for a daily requirement, but protein metabolism isn't regulated daily. It's regulated meal to meal.

Think of protein like water. Let's say the recommendation is to drink eight glasses of water a day. And let's say you drink 80 percent of that amount at night. Well, you're actually dehydrated for most of the day even though you're meeting the daily recommendation. That's not a healthy way to drink. Likewise, you can't make up for lack of protein intake by having a ton at one meal. Instead, hit the protein threshold three to five times a day. If you're a 200-pound guy needing to lose 30 pounds, and you're consuming 140 to 160 grams of protein a day like I recommend, you're going to hit the threshold five times without too much trouble.

A final word about fat before wrapping up my take on diets. Many people assume fat is the most important macronutrient for weight control, but it's not. Certain fats are bad for you, and certain fats are good for you. You have to know which are which. You want to consume those fats that are good for you in relative abundance, even though fat contains 9 calories per gram, 5 more calories than both protein and carbs. You're looking at me crazy, I can tell, but let me explain. Those healthy fats are actually beneficial to your body. What's more, healthy fats make you feel full, discouraging you from eating too many bad fats and simple carbs. So the macronutrient with the most calories can actually help you lose body fat. Trippy concept, huh? Yet it's true.

On my plan, fat intake will be enough to prevent deficiencies in essential fatty acids while optimizing hormone production. Fat will account for 20 percent to 40 percent of caloric intake, depending on total carbs and calories in a given day.

Consuming enough protein is the dietary key to Formula 50. The tissue-building properties of protein are important, the metabolic effect of protein is important, the thermic effect of protein is important, the nutrient-partitioning effect of protein is important, and the body composition effect of protein is important. Protein stimulates all these different things.

The goal is to keep muscle as greedy as possible. In doing so, your muscles will be primed to mercilessly rob calories that might have been destined for your gut or muffin top. That's what is going to keep body fat down for the long term and keep you looking lean and fit.

# 6

# Prepare and Repair: Your Pre- and Post-Workout Tools

**P**HYSICAL PAIN AND I ARE NO STRANGERS. BACK IN 2000, I was unlucky when nine bullets from a 9-millimeter pierced my body in rapid-fire succession. But I was lucky to survive, given that my face and hand were struck, one leg was broken in two places, and the other leg was broken pretty much from hip to knee. My hip also was fractured. I'm lucky I can walk today, let alone work out like I do.

Your brain will survive by any means necessary, and it does so through various protection schemes. For example, in an attempt to keep key organs functioning, the body will respond to trauma by circling the wagons, drawing blood from the extremities into the center of the body. My body did what it could that day to keep enough blood in my body to survive, and I did.

Pain is designed to get your attention. Your body doesn't care about the long term; it's only concerned about right then and there. So let's say you have a hip that doesn't move well, or a tight calf. What's more, you didn't prepare for your workout. Now you're doing a lunge or a squat, but your body has to make adjustments so you don't blow a knee or otherwise get hurt. That dysfunction will accumulate, like a mechanical part of a machine fatiguing over time. One day, all you do is sneeze, and you're like, "Man—I can't move."

What happened? For answers, I spoke with Perry Nickelston, DC, FMS, SFMA, director and owner of Stop Chasing Pain and Fitness 201. He's an expert in how and where movement and pain intersect. Nickelston finds that for patients with, say, knee pain, the solution often lies not in the knee itself but higher or lower than the knee joint. He might show them how to do foam rolling (more on that in a bit) on, or stretching at, their hip joint, or tweak something in their ankle or foot. Suddenly, they're like, "Wow, my knee feels so much better now!" Focusing solely on where the problem expresses itself is like arresting a street hustler on the corner and thinking that'll put his supplier out of business.

I don't fear pain, but I don't seek it out either. Pain isn't a badge of honor; it's a distraction. Back in 2007, I got myself down to 5-percent body fat for the photo shoot for the cover of a CD. Here I was on this motorcycle with a big, heavy chain around my neck and a spinning wheel shooting fire behind me, a scene inspired by Nicolas Cage in *Ghost Rider*. I was dehydrated too. But I sat there all day, holding this damn chain, with the right side of my back having to bear the brunt. The chain was that big. The following day, it was pulling on my left side. Afterward, I ended up going to a chiropractor for electrical stimulation treatments to lessen the discomfort. It helped, but the pain still comes back periodically.

One isolated incident has led to what seems like a lifetime of periodic discomfort. That pain in my back sure has become a pain in my neck.

That's what we want to avoid here. Formula 50 shrinks the chances of you being injured in the first place. Yes, working out and fitness in general help you avoid the injuries that happen when you're sedentary. But you have to be careful. Otherwise, you can harm your body and be sidelined.

Depending on how into fitness you've been up to this point, you may think of it as stuff done with weights, and stuff done on cardio machines. Both activities have something to do with being in shape. You build some muscle with the weights. You increase your endurance on a stair stepper or treadmill. Before either session, maybe you reach down and touch your toes a few times to loosen up, or twist at the trunk while looking in the mirror. Do weights and cardio for long enough, throw in a stretch or two, and you start getting in shape, right?

Well, not so fast. Weights and cardio are important, but another aspect of physical fitness deserves equal weight. I alluded to it a minute ago, but it involves a lot more than doing a few toe touches. This third pillar of fitness *includes* flexibility training, but it really consists of the whole array of things you do a) before your workout to prepare your body and b) after your workout to repair your body. Occasionally you might even do some of this stuff during workouts, although that may get tricky at times during Formula 50. Between-sets rest is in short supply during metabolic resistance training. You may just huff and puff.

Adding pre- and post-workout elements to the mix can make an enormous difference in your entire fitness routine, not to mention in how you feel throughout your day. "I find that people who suffer injuries, from professional athletes down to people who are just living their life—well, the muscular and soft tissue system is seldom looked at as a factor in performance or injury," says Nickelston. "Yet it's a factor with virtually everyone I see."

These aren't the glamour moves of Formula 50. This isn't like hitting a personal best on your bench press or a record time on the treadmill. People often overlook these techniques, or think they're boring, but you need these fundamentals to rise above plateaus and to excel in the other things you want to do as an athlete. These are the supporting strategies that help you achieve major performance gains.

Medicine today is too often about waiting until something is broken and then fixing it. The techniques you'll discover here are about keeping your body from breaking in the first place. You want to be durable, not disposable. Look at LL Cool J—he's had a long, long career (a dozen or so albums for a rap artist!) and a big part of that involves keeping himself in good physical condition. To go the distance like he does, you want to be active and lose weight, but you don't want those efforts to saddle you with aches and pains. You may not feel it as much in your teens and 20s, but in your 30s, 40s, and beyond, look out.

This is a tricky concept because we live in a time of instant gratification. With its youthful audience, hip-hop culture in particular has a short attention span. It's not, "What have you done?" but rather "What have you done for me lately?" But with injury avoidance, it's often, "What did you do to or for your body 2, 5, 10 years ago? How much wear and tear have you inflicted over time?"

If you ignore these preparation and recovery techniques, you might as well be driving your car with the parking break unreleased. You can floor that gas pedal, but you still won't go as fast or as smoothly as you could. So rather than repeatedly pressing that accelerator, you need to figure out how to release the friction holding you back in the first place.

Weights work your skeletal muscles, and cardio works those plus your heart and lungs, but these techniques I'm about to reveal address the connective tissues that hold everything together. The tissues are wrapped around everything from skin to bone, but this interlocking system is often overlooked in medicine and health care. Yet it's something that can be enhanced through the movements we teach you in this book. You'll be amazed how much less pain, stiffness, and tightness you'll feel, how much better you'll move, and how much more quickly you'll burn fat.

What's great about these techniques is that you can learn to do them on your own. In fact, I'm going to teach you to do just that.

## Pre-Workout: Get Ready to Rock

We do most things in a seated position, whether we're sitting at work, sitting in a car, or sitting at home. Even at the gym, sometimes we end up sitting on a machine. Scientists aren't posturing when they claim that all this sitting around is killing us. Unfortunately, Australian researchers recently found that regardless of overall activity levels, people who sit for 11 or more hours a day are 40 percent more likely to die over the next 3 years.

When we do move, whether it's on the treadmill, stair climber, or stationary bike, we tend to move in only one direction: forward. Which is kind of backward.

Like Bob Marley said, get up, stand up—and then move, which is what you'll be doing in my dynamic warm-up drills. You'll be moving not only forward but also backward, left and right, and in different directions. You won't just stride; you'll rotate. Doing 3 or 4 quick drills in this fashion before your workout will give you more benefit and bang for your buck than spending 20 minutes sprawled on a mat doing static stretches. This will prime you for a great workout.

*Activation* is a key word with some of the drills. The goal here is to activate muscles that are normally not active in people, like the gluteus minimus, interscapular muscles, and external rotators. Activating the core is also important. We're trying to switch on certain muscles in your body to prepare them for the challenging moves and physical demands coming their way.

In real life, your body moves in sequences. It has to engage specific muscles at specific times to ensure that you don't fall down. Sometimes we lose that activation ability and muscles don't fire or function as they should. Think of a car with one bad spark plug, and now think of your body with an injury. You have to compensate for that weak link, so you won't move as efficiently as you would have, reducing your metabolic rate. Your injury risk rises because your body now has to compensate for that problem area, where muscles probably aren't "firing." Activation drills are specifically designed to make sure these muscles activate when you want them to—like during the workout to come or when playing a sport.

If you're not used to moving in a certain way, these moves can seem as challenging as the workouts themselves. I've seen high-end athletes drenched in sweat after doing these dynamic warm-ups. Some of these athletes have what I call Ferrari bodies. They look prime and pristine on the outside, but there's only a Volkswagen engine under the hood. All show and no go.

A lot of this stuff comes from rehabilitation science. When Dr. Nickleston welcomes a new patient for some sort of rehab, dynamic warm-ups and activation drills are mandatory. Whether you're an elite athlete or a mom who wants to be able to do activities with her kids, these moves will carry over into every aspect of your life. They're fun and engaging, and they prepare your body for training and life.

These dynamic warm-up moves and activation drills differ from week to week, so they're included in the exercises for each training phase.

# Post-Workout: Apply the Finishing Touches

You finished your last working set and you're totally gassed. Now is the time when you can benefit from stretching.

I know, I know. When you think of stretching, you picture some dude in gym class with a whistle around his neck, telling boys and girls to touch their toes. That's called static stretching, and it's widely misunderstood. Ever notice how everyone doing that looks as stiff as a board? Well, that static stretching isn't effective when done before your body has warmed up. When your body is still cold, static stretching might even be setting you up for the very types of injuries you had hoped to avoid in the first place.

In reality, bending over to touch your toes before your workout is risky. People typically bend at their lower back or lumbar spine instead of at their hips like they should. This increases pressure in their lower back. Do this, and you're actually setting yourself up for a world of hurt, like a bulging or herniated disk, even though you think you're doing something positive.

The problems with static stretching while your body's tissues are cold don't end there. The latest research suggests that static stretching may prompt your nervous system to tell the rest of your body to become tighter, not looser. It's yet another defense mechanism that kicks in when your body senses it's being pushed beyond its limits. *Danger ahead*, says your brain. *Back off. We gotta take precautions.* This is the opposite effect of what you want.

Luckily, stretching and warming up have become more sophisticated, rooted in science rather than misinformation. We now know that it's best to position the static stretching in Formula 50 immediately *after* the workout and before the foam rolling begins. By that point your tissues are warm and elastic; you've already moved your body through various ranges of motion. This reflects the Formula 50 training approach, which favors compound-joint exercises and full-body workouts done at an elevated heart rate.

This is the static stretch sequence you should include at the end of your workouts. I call these moves "static" because you hold the deepest element of the stretch for a period of time, anywhere from 10 to 30 seconds. As I mentioned, this is the time when your body is most warmed up and can benefit the most from stretching. Not only will these stretches help you prevent future injuries or recover from previous ones, but they'll also increase your range of motion.

As a general rule, you want to move into these stretches in a deliberate way with excellent posture and body mechanics. Because you're already warmed up, you can stretch your muscles more deeply at this point. But you don't want to overdo it either. You can push your limits a bit—so long as you don't feel sharp pain or discomfort that's too intense to hold. Back off before either of these occurs.

Avoid dynamic stretching at this point. Don't move in a ballistic way, by using momentum to reach a deeper position. Also, avoid bouncing during your stretches to try to get more extension. While ballistic and dynamic stretching have certain benefits, that's not what I'm emphasizing here. The purpose of these static stretches is to support general fitness and prevent injury.

## Static Stretch Sequence

| Stretch | Target(s) | Reps | Hold Peak Stretch |
| --- | --- | --- | --- |
| 1. Standing Calf | Gastrocnemius | 3/side | 10 seconds |
| 2. Standing Calf | Soleus | 3/side | 10 seconds |
| 3. Standing Quad | Quads | 3/side | 10 seconds |
| 4. Kneeling Hip Flexor | Hip flexors | 3/side | 10 seconds |
| 5. Lying Glutes | Gluteus maxi | 1/side | 30 seconds |
| 6. Lying Hamstrings | Hamstrings | 1/side | 30 seconds |
| 7. Bent-Over Lats | Latissimus dorsi | 3 | 10 seconds |
| 8. Standing Pecs | Pectorals | 3 | 30 seconds |
| 9. Standing Triceps | Triceps | 3/side | 30 seconds |

# Standing Calf

**PURPOSE** | You have two primary calf muscles: the gastrocnemius and the soleus. It's important to target each when you stretch to create better lower leg mobility, faster recovery, and enhanced performance. This stretch targets the "gastroc," the outermost calf muscles at the backs of your lower legs (these are the bulging upside-down heart-shaped muscles you can see from a rearview).

**GET READY** | Stand facing a wall or other vertical support. Place both hands on the support at chest level with your arms fully extended. Move one foot back so that you are in a staggered stance with your feet 2 to 3 feet apart (front to back) and your trailing leg about 3 to 4 feet away from the support. Your body should form a straight line from your back leg through your head. Bend your front leg, and keep your trailing leg in a fully extended position with the entirety of the bottom of your foot contacting the ground.

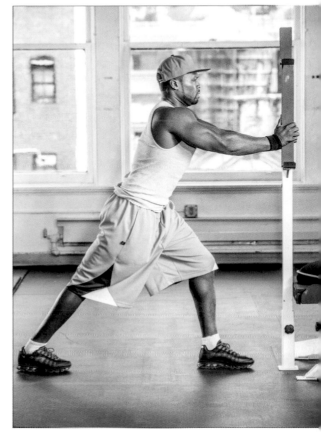

**GO** | Keeping your straight body position from back leg through head, bend your arms, moving your upper body closer to the support, emphasizing a stretch in your gastroc. Make sure the move is slow and deliberate so that you don't bounce and overstretch the muscle. You can perform one long slow stretch, or push in and out of the move, gently testing and stretching the muscle. Then, switch sides and stretch the other-side gastroc.

**FIFTY SAYS** | "If your calves are tight, then you're going to feel this one—and that means you need it. If not, then this stretch is a piece of cake. But you should always include it because effective calf muscle action is crucial for so many moves that don't seem to use them much, such as squats and dead lifts."

## BASIC MOVE
# Standing Calf

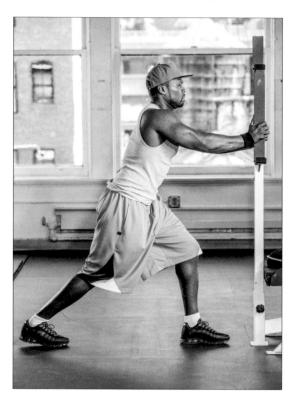

**PURPOSE** | This move, while similar to the other standing calf stretch, has a distinct purpose: This move targets the soleus, the strip of muscle that lies between your tibia and your gastroc. It's visible from both the inner and outer side of each leg. Stretching it is crucial, as it is a major player in lower body activity.

**GET READY** | Stand in front of a wall or other type of vertical support. Place both hands on the support at chest level with your arms fully extended. Step back so you are in a staggered stance with your feet 2 to 3 feet apart (front to back) and your trailing leg about 3 to 4 feet from the support. Bend both knees, keeping the foot of your trailing leg in full contact with the ground.

**GO** | Holding your body position straight from your trailing knee to your head, bend your arms, moving your upper body closer to the supports, emphasizing a stretch in your soleus. The heel of your back foot should maintain full contact with the ground throughout the stretch, and you should maintain the bend in both knees as well. Make sure the move is slow and deliberate so that you don't bounce and overstretch the muscle. You can perform one long slow stretch, or push in and out of the move, gently testing and stretching the muscle. Then, switch sides and stretch the soleus of your other leg.

**FIFTY SAYS** | "Keep in mind that when you're exercising your calves, you always need to work them in a straight-leg and bent-leg position because the straight position activates the gastroc more, and the bent position activates the soleus more. That's true for both muscle-building and stretching."

# Standing Quad

**PURPOSE** | This move helps open and lengthen all your quadriceps muscles.

**GET READY** | Stand facing a wall or other vertical support—you can use a pole for this one since this stretch only requires you to place one hand on the support, and that's more for balance than to hold your body weight (as with the calf stretches). Place one hand on the support, and raise one foot behind you until you can take hold of the top of that foot with your same-side hand. Adjust your body position so that you're standing tall and straight (avoid bending to the side).

**GO** | Gently pull your heel toward your butt, making sure to maintain a tall spine and proper posture. Test how that feels for a couple of seconds. If you can handle a deeper stretch, then gently press your hips forward, allowing your working-side knee to go a bit behind the other knee. Hold that and then repeat on the other side.

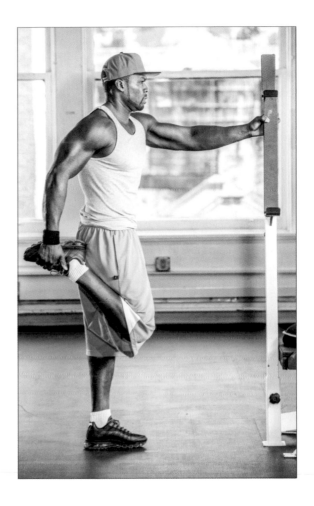

**FIFTY SAYS** | "You probably know that you have tight hamstrings, but you may be surprised to learn that your quads are tight too. When you push your hips forward, you're activating a deeper stretch in your quads than you do in almost any other athletic move. Don't underestimate the benefit of that."

## BASIC MOVE
# Kneeling Hip Flexor

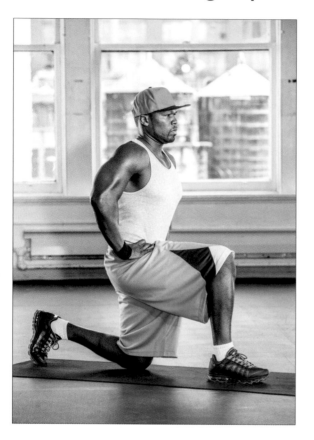

**PURPOSE** | Hip flexors are "minor" lower-body muscles that often cause mobility restrictions. Keeping them stretched out is critical for eliminating a potential weak link in your training.

**GET READY** | With your back knee on the ground, place your front foot on the ground a foot or 2 in front of it. Your lower front leg and upper back leg should be vertical (and parallel). The foot of your lead leg should be flat on the floor, and the toes of your back foot should be in contact with the floor (in other words, don't balance on the top of your trailing foot).

**GO** | Slowly push your hips forward while keeping your torso in an upright position. Also make sure that your hips press forward together—avoid allowing any rotation in your torso. You should feel a stretch in the top of your trailing leg, where your thighs and hips come together. Ease into the position and hold it for several seconds. Then, perform the same move on the other side.

**FIFTY SAYS** | "If this position is uncomfortable, then you can place a towel under your back knee. You should be focused on feeling a stretch in your hip flexors instead of thinking about any pain in your knees."

# Lying Glutes

**PURPOSE** | This stretch not only opens your glutes but it also opens the hips on the other side while you're stretching your working-side glutes. Making sure that you have a flexible glutes/hamstrings tie-in area is one of the keys to avoiding injuries to your backside, a problem many top-tier athletes encounter.

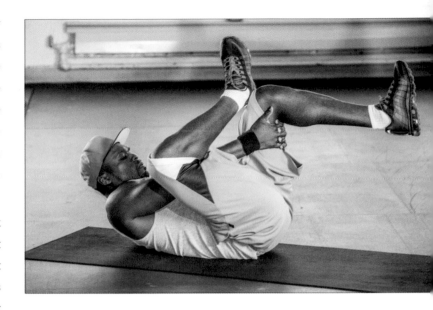

**GET READY** | Lie on your back with your knees bent and your feet flat on the ground. Cross your right leg so that your right ankle rests against your left leg just above that knee. Reaching a hand on either side of your left leg, grasp that leg by the hamstrings, interlocking your fingers if you can. Press your shoulders back and down to the ground, keeping them in that position throughout the stretch.

**GO** | Slowly pull your left leg toward your chest while simultaneously keeping the shin and knee of your right leg perpendicular to your left leg (and parallel to the ground). Relax your shoulders and back into the ground, deepening the stretch. Hold for several seconds, and then repeat on the other side.

**FIFTY SAYS** | "Hard to say where you'll feel this one most—in your glutes on the side that you're holding on to, or in your hip on the other side. That's what makes it such a great stretch."

## BASIC MOVE
# Lying Hamstrings

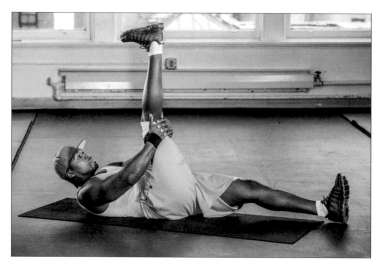

**PURPOSE** | Hamstrings are one of the tightest muscle groups for many men. It's crucial to stretch them, and we've put them last among the lower-body stretches (and particularly after the lying glutes stretch) so that you've had a chance to stretch out the peripheral muscles that may be affecting hamstring flexibility.

**GET READY** | Lie on your back and raise your right leg as high as you can, keeping it straight. Take both hands and interlock them behind your right thigh, if you're able. If not, then bend your knee slightly or place a towel behind your right thigh and grasp it with both hands. Relax your shoulders and back into the ground, and elongate your neck with your head comfortably on the floor.

**GO** | Gently pull your right thigh toward you (using the towel or your hands), making sure that your butt maintains contact with the ground. Avoid twisting—you should feel the same amount of pressure on each of your buttocks. Relax your back, shoulders, neck, and head into the stretch. Focus on keeping your working leg straight and feeling the stretch. Hold, then repeat on other side.

**FIFTY SAYS** | "This is the turbo-charged variation of the lying glutes stretch, and it's a big challenge for a lot of guys. Still, you can take it to the next level by flexing your foot while your leg is straight. To do this, press your straight-leg heel toward the ceiling and angle the toes on that side, a bit, down toward your face."

# Winning the Mind Game

Warming up your body before a workout is important. Never train without having done so. But warming up your muscles and connective tissues is only part of the equation. You also need to prepare your mind for the tasks that lie ahead.

Distractions are everywhere you look in the gym. There's constant motion, dramatic-looking bodies, people doing things that make you want to check them out. I'm not saying you have to train with blinders on, but you do need to keep all this commotion from diluting your focus.

The key is to make sure this mind-set is established before you start working out. All great athletes and performers do this. They don't just wander out into the arena and say, "Oh, wow, let's get after it." They're ready from the jump-off because they focused beforehand.

Here are three tips to help you get into a zone and stay there for your whole workout:

1. On the drive to the gym, go through your workout in your mind. Actually picture yourself nailing each set with perfect form. By the time the workout starts, you'll simply be giving a repeat performance of a great workout.

2. When you arrive at the gym, take everything that's been troubling you, put it in an imaginary box, and set it aside, as if you were dropping something off at the front desk. It will still be there when your workout is done, but it won't sidetrack you.

3. Listen to music when you train, and I say that not just because I'm a musician. Music does at least two things. First, the headphones will tell people you mean business. Second, music can inspire you to make a better effort. We all know the feelings music evokes in our body, even if we're driving and a great song comes on. Use that to your advantage in the gym by programming your iPod with stuff that sends your brain and central nervous system into overdrive.

## BASIC MOVE
# Bent-Over Lats

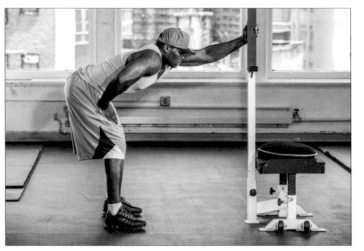

**PURPOSE** | To open the shoulder joint and, particularly, to stretch the lats, especially where they attach along the sides of your body. Having more flexible lats allows for a more open hands-over-head position for pressing and pulling moves, making it easier to more effectively work your shoulders and back.

**GET READY** | Stand in front of a solid horizontal surface at about hip-to-navel height—a Smith machine or racked barbell set to this height are good options. Take hold of the bar with your hands spaced at about shoulder-width. Step back from the bar so that you will be able to bend over with your legs perpendicular to the ground and your arms straight (you can work into this as the stretch progresses). Your torso should be about parallel to the floor (or a little higher if you're less flexible). Bend your knees if needed to allow you to get your upper body in the proper position.

**GO** | Maintaining the natural curve in your lower back, slowly shift your hips to the left while keeping a firm grip on the bar. You should feel a stretch along the right side of your upper body as you create a small arch along that side. Then shift your hips to the right.

**FIFTY SAYS** | "This is another one that just feels so right when you do it. I like to do this stretch in between sets too."

# Standing Pecs

**PURPOSE** | Most guys have tight pecs, and they don't even know it. This comes from allowing the shoulders to roll forward, especially during activities such as working at a keyboard. This chest stretch is critical for helping to stretch out the pecs and open the shoulder joint.

**GET READY** | Face into a doorway if one of the proper width for you is available in your gym—if not, then perform the stretch one side at a time, using a doorframe or upright post (or perform the corner stretch, described below). Bend your arms at a 90-degree angle at the elbows, and place your forearms against the sides of the doorframes. Your upper arms should be parallel to the ground and in line with your shoulders, and your lower arms should point upward with palms on the doorframe.

**GO** | Step forward with one foot, allowing your chest to arch from side to side. Pull in your abs a bit to put more of the stretch into your pectorals. Hold this for 30 seconds, then ease out of it, rest for a few seconds, and then repeat.

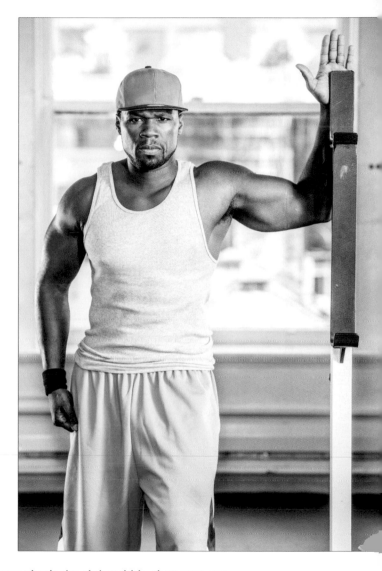

**FIFTY SAYS** | "If you can't find a doorframe that's the right width, then you can also perform this by facing into a corner. In fact, I like to use both a doorway and a corner because you get a slightly different feel from each. And, trust me, you probably need more flexibility in your pecs."

## BASIC MOVE
# Standing Triceps

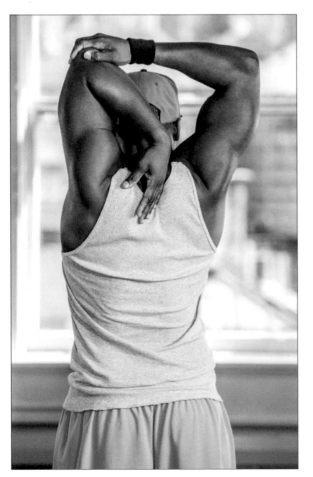

**PURPOSE** | To stretch your triceps and open up your shoulder joint.

**GET READY** | While standing, raise your left arm above your head and bend it at the elbow so that your left hand is touching your upper back between your shoulder blades. Take your right arm and reach up and take hold of your left arm just above the elbow.

**GO** | Gently press against your left arm with your right, taking the upper portion of your working-side arm as low as you comfortably can. Hold the stretch position for several seconds, then repeat on the other side.

**FIFTY SAYS** | "You can also perform this move by placing your upper arm against a doorframe or vertical post. Then, lean gently into it, allowing the frame or post to stretch your triceps and open your shoulder."

## Foam Rolling Stretches

Foam rollers are relative newcomers to the gym. They've been around since the 1990s, but they've grown in popularity. Now, they're standard fare at most gyms. You can also buy one for home. This sequence is a great rest day "workout," and it will help you recover faster from your other strenuous workouts.

Before you buy a roller for home, though, you should try one at the gym to see what type you like best. Foam rollers come in various densities—from those with plenty of "give" to those that are rock solid, allowing you to work deeply into the muscle.

In the Formula 50 foam rolling sequence, you'll hit 8 knot-prone areas, from calves to spine. You'll spend 30 seconds on each area—more if you find a sore or tender spot. If you don't feel any, that's great, but spend 30 seconds on that muscle anyway. Trigger points will sting when you hit them, but this shouldn't feel like you're water-boarding yourself with Styrofoam. In fact, the body tends to pull back and shut down if something becomes too painful for too long.

The foam rolling stretches apply passive pressure, which helps relax your muscles as external force is applied. They also actively engage your muscles, stretching them at the end of your workouts. By loyally following this foam rolling sequence at the end of your workouts, you'll recover more quickly and be more open and flexible for the other exercises in future workouts.

Whether you want to roll on an off day or on cardio-only days is up to you. If you're rehabilitating an injury, daily foam rolling probably makes sense. Otherwise, I'd give your body a break from rolling on non-weight-training days. Once you become adept at rolling, 3 or 4 days a week should work best.

# Foam Rolling Stretch Sequence

| Stretch | Target(s) | Minimum Roll Time |
| --- | --- | --- |
| 1. Calves Foam Roll | Calves | 30 seconds per side |
| 2. Hamstrings Foam Roll | Hamstrings | 30 seconds per side |
| 3. Glutes Foam Roll | Glutes | 30 seconds per side |
| 4. IT Band Foam Roll | IT band | 30 seconds per side |
| 5. Quads Foam Roll | Quads | 30 seconds per side |
| 6. Adductors Foam Roll | Adductors | 30 seconds per side |
| 7. Lats Foam Roll | Lats | 30 seconds per side |
| 8. Spine Foam Roll | Spine, back, traps | 60 seconds |

BASIC MOVE

## BASIC MOVE
# Calves Foam Roll

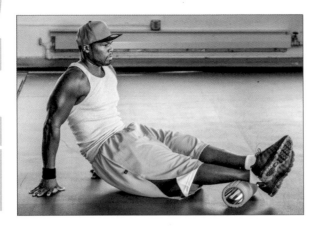

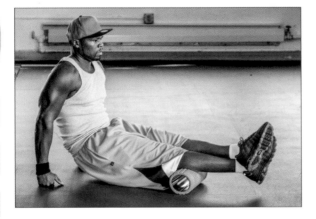

**PURPOSE** | To apply deep pressure to the gastroc and soleus, the primary muscles of your calves.

**GET READY** | Sit on the ground and place the roller under your right calf. Place the palms of your hands on the ground with your thumbs pointing toward your feet. Place your left leg on top of your right (to get it out of the way and to add more weight to your working leg).

**GO** | Raise your butt so only your hands are touching the ground. Keeping your chest up and your spine in proper alignment, roll back and forth with your calf in a neutral position. Then externally rotate your lower leg so that you can roll on to the outer muscles (including the soleus). Next, rotate your lower leg in and roll the inner portion of the muscle. Then do the same on the other leg.

**FIFTY SAYS** | "Calves are a tricky muscle group, and rolling them out will keep them from getting tight or injured."

# Hamstrings Foam Roll

**PURPOSE** | This roll helps reduce tightness and sore points on the backsides of your upper legs and encourages more range of motion.

**GET READY** | Sit on the ground with the roller under your right thigh. Place your knuckles on the ground with your thumbs pointing toward your feet. You can place your left leg on top of the right to get it out of the way and add a little weight while you're rolling.

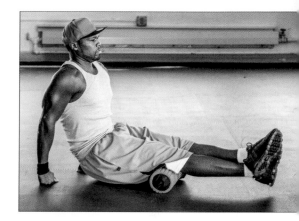

**GO** | Raise your butt so only your hands are touching the ground. Keeping your chest up and your spine in proper alignment, roll back and forth with your hamstrings in a neutral position. Allow the foam roller to move under you from the bottom of your hipbone to the top of your knees. After you've rolled from top to bottom a few times, externally rotate your leg a bit so that the outer portion of your hamstrings contacts the roller. Perform a couple rolls in this position, and then turn your leg so that you can roll the inner portion of your hamstrings. Then repeat the process with the other leg.

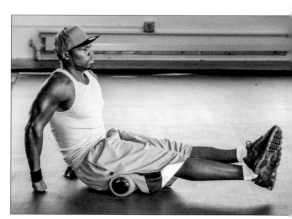

**FIFTY SAYS** | "This one feels really good, especially at the top of the roll. I like to do this on a firm roller to really penetrate into the thick muscle tissue."

# Glutes Foam Roll

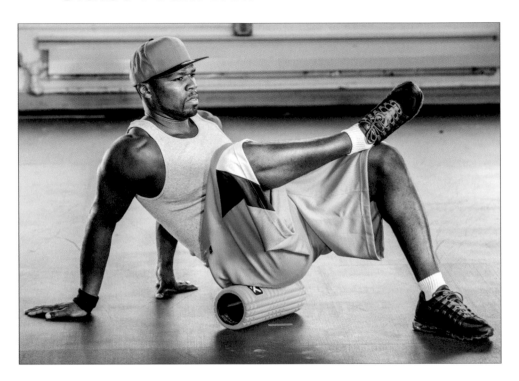

**PURPOSE** | To penetrate deeply into the thick gluteal tissue to reach any knots or tight areas. Increased flexibility in the glutes also helps increase range of motion for hamstrings work such as stiff-leg dead lifts, Romanian dead lifts, and hyperextensions.

**GET READY** | Sit on the roller with just one of your glutes contacting it. Cross the leg on that side and rest that foot on your opposite knee. Lean on your butt so that the working side of your body is angled down toward the ground. Place your hand or forearm behind you on the ground.

**GO** | Roll your gluteal muscles from your hipbone to just below your lower back. You can allow the leg of your non-working side to touch the ground, if necessary, to assist with balance. Then repeat on the other side.

**FIFTY SAYS** | "Relax your butt. That's the key to this roll. The tightness is usually deep, so you have to let your butt muscles go to reach the problem areas."

# IT Band Foam Roll

**PURPOSE** | Your IT (iliotibial) band is a thick bunch of connective tissue that runs along the outside of your thigh, and it is often a source of extreme tightness or pain. Rolling and stretching it are extremely beneficial in making certain that it is not a limiting factor in your training.

**GET READY** | Lie on your side and place the foam roller underneath your lower thigh, just above the joint of your knee, and extend your working leg until it's straight. Cross your other (upper) leg over your lower (working) leg. Place your hands on the ground in a way that will allow you to move the roller from just above your knee to your upper thigh.

**GO** | Pressing through your arms and using your upper body muscles, slowly roll up and down your outer thigh from just above your knee to below your hipbone. Position yourself on the other side and repeat.

**FIFTY SAYS** | "This is overlooked by many people, but it's an important hot spot for tightness and trigger points. Resist the temptation to skip it."

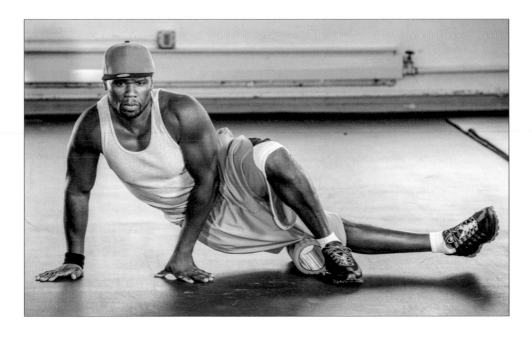

## BASIC MOVE
# Quads Foam Roll

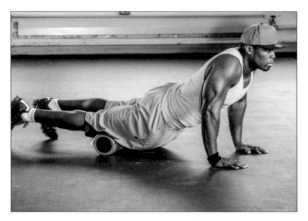

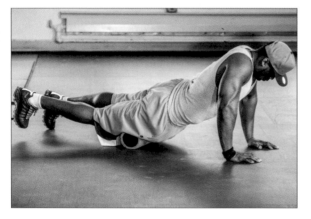

**PURPOSE** | To roll out tension and tightness in your quads.

**GET READY** | Lie facedown with your right thigh in contact with the foam roller. The roller should contact your quads just above your kneecap. Place your hands or forearms on the ground for balance. Lift your left leg off the ground; only the toes of your left foot should touch the ground.

**GO** | Supporting your body weight with your hands or forearms, roll up and down from the top of your knee to the bottom of your hipbone. After you've rolled your leg in the neutral position a few times, turn your leg in to roll your inner quads. Then turn your leg outward and roll the outer quads. When you've finished with these variations, then roll the quads of your other leg.

**FIFTY SAYS** | "Man, this roll is intense, especially at the top of the quads. I like to use a slightly softer foam roller for this one, especially when my quads are sore from a workout from the day before."

# Adductors Foam Roll

**PURPOSE** | The adductors are inner thigh muscles that run from your inner knee up into your groin, and groin injuries are legendary. This roll will help prevent these athletic injuries and warn you of any impending problems based on tightness.

**GET READY** | For this move, turn the roller 90 degrees compared to the preceding rolls so that it will roll side to side instead of up and down your body. Get on top of the roller, facing down, and place your hands or forearms on the ground. Adjust the roller so that it contacts the inside of one leg near the knee. Your opposite, non-working leg should contact the ground for balance. Your working leg should be comfortably bent at the knee.

**GO** | Roll the apparatus from the top of your knee up into your groin, applying as much pressure as you can—tight hips may prevent you from applying deep pressure as you approach your groin. Adjusting your non-working leg will allow you to intensify or lessen the amount of pressure applied to the target muscle. Spend equal time on each leg.

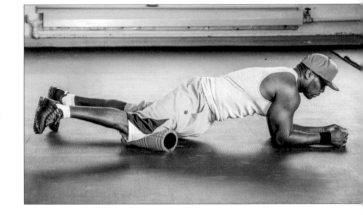

**FIFTY SAYS** | "You may get some strange looks when you're performing this one, but it's important for preventing injury and helping you to open your hips for other athletic moves."

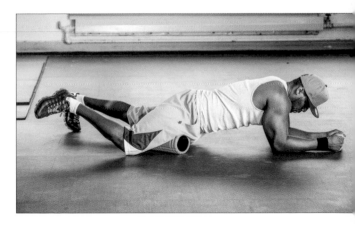

## BASIC MOVE
# Lats Foam Roll

**PURPOSE** | The sides of your lats are often overlooked in training and stretching—in fact, even many masseuses forget to work the portion of your lats that wrap around and connect to the sides of your body. As such, you may find that this is a particularly tender area, which is an indication of how important it is to roll them out.

**GET READY** | Lie across the foam roller with it contacting your side just below your pectoral muscles. Your body should be in a side-plank position. Straighten your (lower) working-side arm along the floor to open your lats. Place your feet comfortably on the floor for balance.

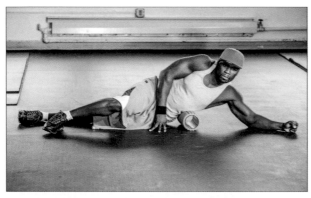

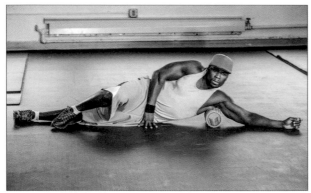

**GO** | Roll just past your shoulder and armpit, and then back to your pecs. As you roll, experiment with tilting your torso slightly forward or back to zero in on tender spots. When you tilt the front of your body toward the ground, you'll hit your pectoral muscles; when you tilt the backside of your body toward the ground, you'll hit some of the smaller muscles of your back and shoulders, all of which tend to be tight. Give equal time to each side.

**FIFTY SAYS** | "As with your IT band, many people find this area to be very tender. This foam rolling move will help iron out these knots."

# Spine Foam Roll

**PURPOSE** | This move helps open up your thoracic ("T") spine, the portion between your neck and lower back. This is a critical roll for improving general posture and reducing "hunching." Poor posture undercuts athletic performance and increases the risk of injury.

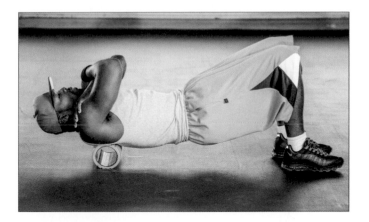

**GET READY** | Lie on your back with the foam roller placed at your mid-back. Cross your arms over your chest as if you're giving yourself a hug (place each hand on your opposite side to open your back more from side to side). Place your feet on the floor with knees bent. At this point only your feet should be in contact with the ground.

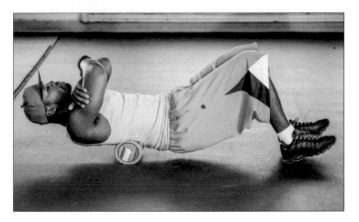

**GO** | Roll up toward the top of your back, stopping before you reach your neck. Then roll back down to your mid-back. As you get more accustomed to this move, you can change your hand positions to target your back muscles in slightly different ways. Extend your arms overhead and roll, and extend your arms out to your sides and roll.

**FIFTY SAYS** | "If you sit in front of a computer all day, this one is going to feel really good. The T spine often becomes hunched from sitting in front of a computer, and this is a major cause of neck and shoulder pain."

## Massage: Weighing the Benefits

As long as you secure the services of a skilled practitioner who understands the systems of the body, massage can be a very effective recuperation technique. I'd go as far as to say that massage is one of the best tools in the business for recovery and regeneration. For elite athletes, it's mandatory. But even if you just want to feel good and stay fit, a nice targeted or general massage can help release tension from your body and take the weight from your mind.

The type of massage you go for is up to you. It depends on the practitioner's skill and technique. Massage is an art form; some people just have that gift. Find somebody whose touch fits well with your body. With something like a deep tissue sports massage, you'll just have to see if you can tolerate it, because it can be painful. But we're not talking about going on a cruise ship and getting a spa massage here. You want something that can help your body recover and enhance your performance.

# 7

# Formula 50, the Beginner Plan

**T**HEY SAY IT TAKES 30 DAYS TO MAKE A HABIT. IF YOU'RE a drug addict in a 12-step program, the 30-day mark becomes a monumental threshold for that reason: The old unhealthy ways need to be replaced by healthier ways. The same threshold applies if you're trying to go from out of shape to in shape. Thirty days. A little more than 4 weeks. Stick with it for that long, and your odds for success skyrocket.

Those adjustments make the first 30 days the most challenging. Go to any gym at the top of the year, and it'll be packed with people acting on New Year's resolutions. Everybody wants to change, even if it's to lose 4 pounds or take a little pinch off their paunch. Guys who are smaller are trying to bulk up, and some of the bigs want to shrink it down. Supplement stores and websites always see a big spike at this time of year. People seem committed. But most end up quitting early on.

Just stick with me for 30 days.

During the beginner's phase of Formula 50, you'll be doing 3 days of total-body metabolic resistance training and 2 days of interval training (or what we call energy system training). Then you'll be taking 2 days off from dedicated workouts, although I encourage you to be active on those days. Go for a walk with your guy or girl, head to the beach, play some touch football, whatever. I encourage that. For beginners, this 3-and-2-plus-active-rest approach works wonders at changing body composition.

You might be thinking, *But Fifty—I'm ready to rock this. I'm ready to hit the weights 7 days a week if that's what it takes.* I appreciate that sentiment, but that's *not* what it takes. That mind-set can set the stage for failure rather than success. How much exercise have you undertaken over the last few months? Be honest. Nothing? Okay, so you're going to go from doing nothing to doing something every damn day? That's a huge change, one that very few people are able to sustain.

Avoid becoming too ambitious too fast. We live in a culture where people expect results right away, and that's not always possible, especially with fitness. Good things are happening inside you all the while, but it takes several weeks to start seeing significant adaptations from exercise, so it's very important to set realistic goals. Better to be pleasantly surprised when you exceed them rather than disillusioned if you fall short.

An all-or-nothing mentality makes people give up when problems arise. Perfect is the enemy of good, as they say. People think, *Well, I missed one workout, so now all is lost.* The setbacks also can be physical as well as mental when you try to progress too quickly or pick up immediately from where you left off a few years ago, as if you had never even stopped. If your body isn't given enough time to recover, injuries happen. And when they do, you may think: *Well, maybe exercise isn't for me.*

Just stick with me for 30 days.

Hitting the weights three times a week at first should be manageable. You'll get used to preparing for your workouts. This might mean packing your gym bag the night before, getting used to going to the gym before or on the way home from work, or training on your lunch break. Regardless, good habits will form, and bad habits will begin to fade.

Goal setting is critical for staying the course. Your initial goal might just be *I will exercise consistently*. You don't need to be lifting as much as the biggest guy in the gym, sprinting faster than everyone else on the treadmill, or sprouting new muscles overnight. The goal is simply to show up for and then complete each workout.

Henry Ford, founder of the car company, said something to the effect that every large undertaking is easy if you break it down into small jobs. Hence the assembly line approach to automobile making. Sculpting your body is no different from assembling chassis. Set smaller steps that add up to bigger achievements.

Much of the initial work in Formula 50 involves body-weight exercises to develop core stability and enhance mobility in the thoracic spine and hips. Once those have been improved, we can start increasing intensity en route to the results you're after.

Some of you may feel like you want to shape up, that you're ready to change. At the same time, joining a gym might seem intimidating. After all, the gym can seem threatening and alien. Find a health club where you feel comfortable. If you're unsure, most places will give you a pass for a few days or a week. Don't just waltz in on a Saturday afternoon and think, *Wow, this is great. Nobody's here!* Visit at the times that you would actually use it, like Monday and Tuesday before or after work.

Sticking with the diet during the first few weeks of any program is almost always challenging. Keep your expectations realistic. Research has shown that people can safely and effectively lose 1 to 2 pounds a week. That may not seem like a lot until you realize that each of those fat pounds represents 3,500 calories of energy. So if you're 100 pounds overweight, and each of those pounds equals 3,500 calories, that's 350,000 calories you need to ditch just to get back to normal. That's a big hole you've dug for yourself with a fork and spoon.

We're going to dig you out of it through higher energy expenditure with lower intake. You have a number of fat-burning tools at your disposal in Formula 50. They'll all work together to help you achieve your goal. First, the workouts will increase your energy expenditure, perhaps dramatically, depending on what you're doing now. You'll also be making smarter food choices. You'll be planning ahead, reading food labels, understanding what a serving size means, and so on. A lot of people don't realize that products they perceive as healthy—say, a bottle of fruit juice—can be gut bombs. That bottle of juice may have more than 100 calories per serving, and a 20-ounce bottle could contain 2½ servings.

# Tools You'll Need to Transform

Here are some of the things I want you focus on during these first few weeks:

*Intensity*: This term is used several ways in a workout context, starting with how hard you train. For you beginners, we're using a rating of perceived exertion scale. Basically it assigns a score to how hard you think you're working, rather than taking some more objective measurement like heart rate. The scale ranges from 1, which is about as taxing as picking up a newspaper, to 10, the sort of Herculean effort that'll make you feel like an ant carrying 50 times its body weight. (They can.) A typical workout intensity might register at a 6, which is equal to around 65 or 70 percent of your max effort.

As long as you build up to it, higher intensity is a good thing. All these workouts are total body and metabolic. Over time, your rest periods are shortened, increasing the energy demands and forcing you to adapt. You couldn't have handled the rest periods of, say, Week 6, which are only 15 seconds, in Week 1. But most likely you can handle the 60 seconds you were given in Week 1. Again, gradual improvement is the key.

*Form:* If you're a rank beginner, the most important thing to do is ace your form. Until your form is tight, you shouldn't be doing the aerobic half of these moves at anything approaching, say, 9 on a scale of 1 to 10. You might do a 6, like some light jogging in place, and then try to build up from there. This strategy seems to work well for beginners. As you do with all physical fitness, you acclimate to the training.

## Phase 1: Weeks 1–2

During the first 2 weeks, the objective is to improve aerobic power and body composition. You'll be training five times a week and resting the other 2 days.

Pick your preferred cardio mode. It doesn't have to be the stationary bike. It could be boxing, rowing, running, or cycling. Just as long as you get that heart and those lungs pumping. The volume and rest intervals will vary over the 6 weeks.

| Week | Monday | Tuesday | Wednesday | Thursday | Friday | Saturday | Sunday |
|---|---|---|---|---|---|---|---|
| #1 | Strength 1 | EST 1 | Strength 1 | EST 1 | Strength 1 | Off | Off |
| #2 | Strength 1 | EST 1 | Strength 1 | EST 1 | Strength 1 | Off | Off |

EST = Energy System Training

### EST 1

**Warm-up:** 5 minutes on treadmill at leisurely pace.

**Intervals:** Do 3 to 5 per session. If you can't manage to do 5 in Week 1, try to reach 5 by the end of Week 2. Make that your goal. Each interval should last 3 minutes at an intensity that feels somewhat hard. Follow up each of these work intervals with 1 minute done at an intensity that feels moderate. This is the rest interval. So start to finish, not counting that 5-minute warm-up, the interval session should last 12 to 18 minutes, depending on whether you complete 3, 4, or 5 intervals.

**Cool-down:** 5 minutes on treadmill at leisurely pace.

## STRENGTH 1

### Dynamic Warm-Up/Flexibility

| Exercise | Sets | Reps | Load | Tempo | Rest | Intensity |
|---|---|---|---|---|---|---|
| Side-Lying Spinal Twist | 1 | 5/side | Body-weight | Moderate | None | Low |
| Lying Knee Drop | 1 | 5/side | Body-weight | Moderate | None | Low |
| Hip Flexor Stretch | 1 | 5/side | Body-weight | Moderate | None | Low |
| Walking Lunge Stretch | 1 | 5/side | Body-weight | Moderate | None | Low |

### Activation Drills

| Drill | Sets | Reps | Load | Tempo[1] | Rest | Intensity |
|---|---|---|---|---|---|---|
| Hip Bridge | 1 | 10–12 | Body-weight | 2011 | None | Low |
| Standing Y-Raise | 1 | 10 | Body-weight | 2011 | None | Low |

### Strength Training

| Exercise | Sets[2] | Reps | Load[3] | Tempo[1] | Rest (secs) | Intensity |
|---|---|---|---|---|---|---|
| A1. Split Squat | 3 | 10–12/side | TBD | 2110 | 60, 45 | Moderate |
| A2. Push-Up | 3 | To failure | TBD | 2010 | 60, 45 | Moderate |
| B1. Hip Thrust | 3 | 10–12 | TBD | 2011 | 60, 45 | Moderate |
| B2. Lat Pull-Down | 3 | 10–12 | TBD | 3010 | 60, 45 | Moderate |
| C1. Biceps Curl | 3 | 10–12 | TBD | 3010 | 60, 45 | Moderate |
| C2. Rear Delt Raise | 3 | 10–12 | TBD | 2011 | 60, 45 | Moderate |
| D1. Plank | 3 | 30 seconds | Body-weight | Hold | 60, 45 | Moderate |

[1] "Tempo" refers to the speed of movement. For example, 3-1-1-0 means: 3 seconds lowering the weight; 1 second pause in the lengthened position; 1 second to raise the weight; no pause ("0") in the contracted position.

[2] When you see exercises preceded by the same letter, complete these sets before moving on to the next pairing. For example, do a set of split squats (A1), rest 60 seconds, do a set of push-ups (A2), rest 60 seconds, and then do another set of split squats. Only after finishing all 3 sets for each of those exercises do you proceed to the next pairing (B, in this case). Perform those paired sets in the same fashion. In week 2, reduce rest to 45 seconds.

[3] Choose a weight that allows you to fail in the desired rep range. For the biceps curl, if you can do only 7 reps, your weight is too heavy. If you can do 13, it's too light.

**Flexibility training:** Perform immediately post-workout. See Chapter 6, page 61, for details.

**Foam rolling:** Perform immediately after stretching. See Chapter 6, page 72, for details.

## DYNAMIC WARM-UP/FLEXIBILITY
### BASIC MOVE
# Side-Lying Spinal Twist

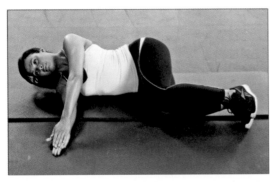

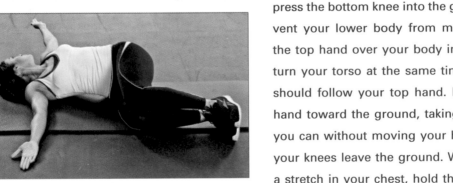

**PURPOSE** | To open upper and lower back to increase mobility, and to warm up muscles to prevent injury.

**GET READY** | Lie on your side with your legs bent at about 90 degrees. Extend your arms in front of you, in line with your shoulders, with your hands together.

**GO** | Squeeze your knees together and press the bottom knee into the ground to prevent your lower body from moving. Rotate the top hand over your body in an arch and turn your torso at the same time. Your eyes should follow your top hand. Move the top hand toward the ground, taking it as low as you can without moving your hips or letting your knees leave the ground. When you feel a stretch in your chest, hold the position for a second, and then return to the starting position. With each repetition, you should be able to move your top shoulder and hand a little closer to the ground. Perform all repetitions on one side and then switch to the other.

**FIFTY SAYS** | "This move just feels good, whether you perform it at the beginning, middle, or end of your workouts. It's great for opening up your back."

# Lying Knee Drop

**PURPOSE** | To open your hips and warm up your knee and ankle joints.

**GET READY** | Lie on your back and bend your legs, placing your feet on the floor wider than your hips. Put your arms out to your sides, palms facing the ceiling.

**GO** | Exhale and drop your left knee inward, toward the center of your body, as far as you can without allowing your hip to come off the floor. Make sure your foot stays flat on the floor as you move your knee. Pause, and then bring that knee back to the start position. Perform the same movement with your right knee. Alternate legs until you've performed the prescribed reps.

**FIFTY SAYS** | "This is a unique way to warm up the joints of your lower extremities—great for prepping for heavier weight moves like lunges and squats."

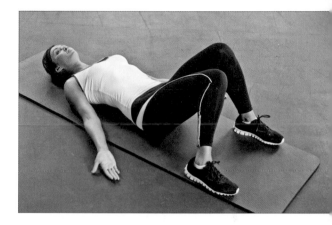

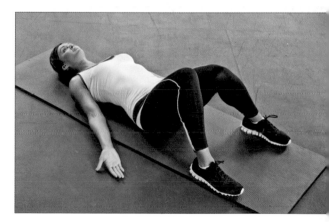

# Hip Flexor Stretch

**PURPOSE** | To stretch upper legs, core, and shoulders while getting a total-body warm-up.

**GET READY** | Put a mat on the ground and place your right knee on the mat under your right hip with your right foot bent and your toes on the ground. Place your left foot a couple feet in front of your body, with your left leg bent 90 degrees.

**GO** | Keeping your chest up, raise your arms over your head. Press your right knee into the ground and shift your hips forward, maintaining an upright body position. Feel the stretch in your right hip flexor, pause for a second, and then ease back to the starting position. Perform all reps on this side before moving onto the other.

**FIFTY SAYS** | "Great way to open your hip joints. When I raise my hands over-head, it opens the whole front side of my body."

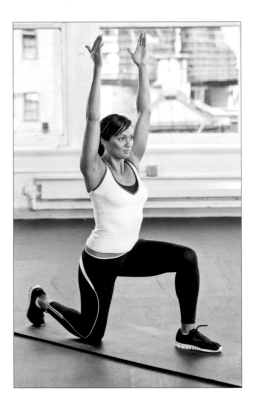 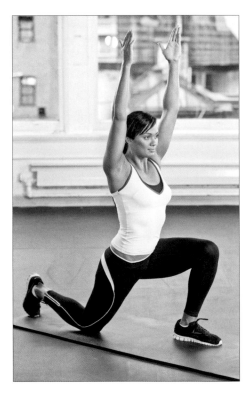

# Walking Lunge Stretch

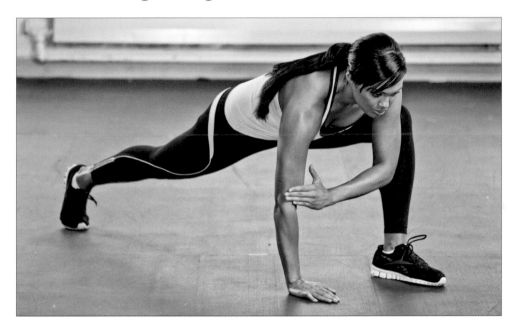

**PURPOSE** | To warm you up for the more challenging weighted lunges you'll perform later in the workout.

**GET READY** | Stand tall with your feet hip-width apart and chest out.

**GO** | Step forward with your left foot, placing it as far out as you comfortably can. Come up onto the toes of your trailing leg and lower your hips. Put your right hand firmly on the floor, and then, keeping your chest up and your back leg straight, drive your left elbow down toward your left foot. Feel the stretch in your groin as you pause for a second; then step your trailing leg forward, standing upright. Next, step the other leg forward and continue moving across the floor until you've completed all reps for each side.

**FIFTY SAYS** | "This is a dynamic stretch that's great after you've performed some of the more basic stretches in my warm-up."

## ACTIVATION DRILLS

**BASIC MOVE**

# Hip Bridge

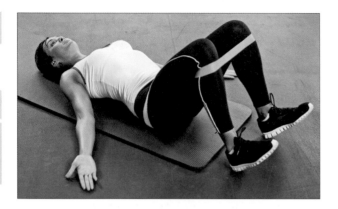

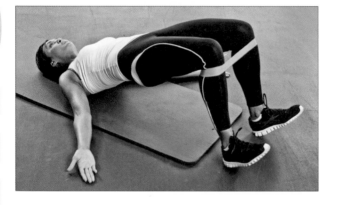

**PURPOSE** | This stretch uses a mini-band to hold your knees together, adding tension to hip thrusts.

**GET READY** | Wrap a mini-band around both legs, just below your knees, and lie on your back with your knees bent. Place your feet flat on the floor and angle your arms out from your body with your palms facing up to help anchor you during the move.

**GO** | Pull your toes up toward your shins so your heels are the only part of your feet that contacts the floor. Press your legs outward slightly to create tension against the mini-band. Raise your hips off the floor and squeeze your glutes so that your knees, hips, and shoulders form a straight line. Pause at the top for about 2 seconds, and then slowly lower to the starting position.

**FIFTY SAYS** | "You can shift your foot position an inch or 2 closer or farther away from your butt between sets so that you get a slightly different stretch each time."

# Standing Y-raise

**PURPOSE** | To warm up and open your shoulders for the upper-body moves to come in the strength-training portion of this workout.

**GET READY** | Place your feet shoulder distance apart and bend at the hips until your upper body forms a 45-degree angle with the floor. You can bend a bit at the knees to make this angle more comfortable. Let your arms hang at your sides, perpendicular to the ground, with your thumbs facing forward and palms open toward each other.

**GO** | Hold your shoulder blades back and down, then raise your arms until they form a straight line with your torso. Allow your arms to open out a little bit so that they form a "Y" with your upper body. Keep all movements slow and deliberate, performing the prescribed number of reps.

**FIFTY SAYS** | "If you have tight shoulders, you can also perform this stretch with your chest pressed into an incline bench to give you a little leverage."

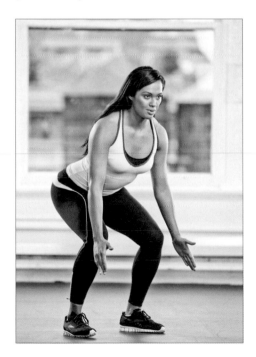
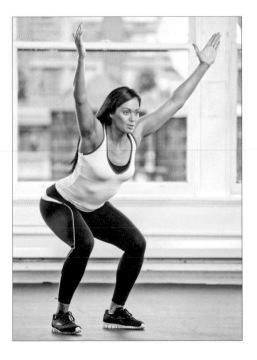

## STRENGTH TRAINING

**BASIC MOVE**

# Split Squat

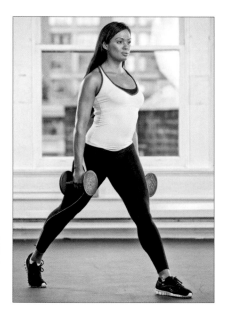

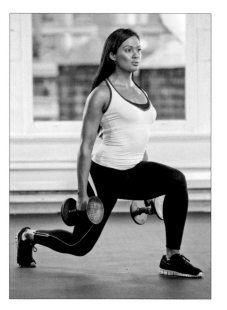

**SPECIAL FEATURES** | Dumbbell, stationary, non-alternating

**TARGET** | Legs, glutes

**PURPOSE** | This move works the front and back of your legs differently, targeting the quads, glutes, and hamstrings in two unique ways. It also requires you to stabilize your core to maintain your balance.

**GET READY** | Hold a pair of dumbbells with your hands at your waist, palms facing each other.

**GO** | Keeping the natural curve in your back and remaining fully upright with your chest out, stride forward with one foot. Place that foot flat on the ground. Lower your body until your back knee comes close to the ground, allowing your back heel to leave the ground. Try not to let your back knee strike the ground. Then, driving through your front foot and keeping your glutes engaged and torso perpendicular to the ground, step back until you are upright. Perform all reps on this side before repeating on the other.

**FIFTY SAYS** | "Lunges may look easy, but they require a lot of balance and strength. You can make them even harder by progressively increasing the length of your stride."

# Push-Up

**SPECIAL FEATURES** | Standard

**TARGET** | Primarily the pectorals but also the triceps and shoulders

**PURPOSE** | When performed correctly, push-ups provide a great stretch and flex for the pectorals, making them stronger for increased muscle mass and muscular endurance.

**GET READY** | Get into the top of a push-up position, with hands placed slightly wider than your shoulders. Place your feet about hip-distance apart, putting your weight on your toes. Keep your head in its natural alignment by looking at the ground throughout the set.

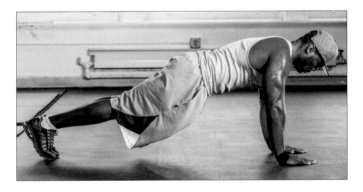

**GO** | Lower your body close to the floor by bending at the elbows and keeping the rest of your body, from head to toes, in one line. Feel the stretch in your pecs as you hover just above the ground. With control, press back up. Keep your shoulders back and shoulder blades pulled together

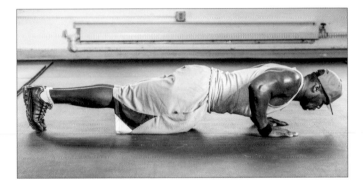

to emphasize the work in your pecs. Don't allow your back to round side to side at the top of the movement. Feel a contraction in your chest at the top of the movement, and then perform the next rep.

**FIFTY SAYS** | "The goal isn't to do as many push-ups as your ego demands but to perform each rep with the best form possible to maximize chest development."

## BASIC MOVE

# Hip Thrust

**SPECIAL FEATURES** | Weighted, barbell

**TARGET** | Legs, glutes, core

**PURPOSE** | To develop core strength as you work your legs and midsection in a unique way.

**GET READY** | Place your upper back and shoulders on the edge of a bench and slide your hips under a barbell—use light, rubber, or plastic weights to elevate the barbell until you're able to perform the move with 45-pound plates (you can add smaller

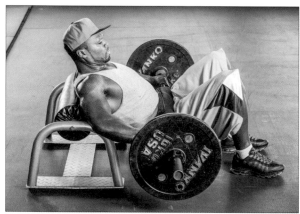

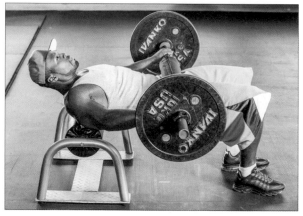

weights to the light "holder" plates). To assume the starting position, place your feet on the floor and bend at the knees so that your upper and lower legs form a 45-degree angle. Balance the barbell on your hips, holding it in place with your hands.

**GO** | With your body secure and your core tight, press your heels into the floor. Contract your glutes and hamstrings, and then press your hips up until your body forms a line, from knees to head, that's parallel to the floor. Protect your back by maintaining its neutral alignment throughout the set. Hold the weight at the top for a second, and then lower the weight with control until your glutes touch the ground.

**FIFTY SAYS** | "This move is a little tricky at first, but it's a great way to work your core, glutes, and legs."

# Lat Pull-Down

**SPECIAL FEATURES** | Underhand grip

**TARGET** | Latissimus dorsi (lats)

**PURPOSE** | To increase mass and detail of the largest back muscles.

**GET READY** | Adjust the load of a pull-down machine to a weight that allows you to perform the desired number of reps. (Finding the right amount of weight may require experimentation.) Take hold of the bar with an underhand grip (palms facing your body), hands shoulder-distance apart. Pull the bar lower so that you can secure your thighs under the leg pads.

**GO** | Begin the motion by pinching your scapula together and then pulling the weight toward your chest. Hold your back in its neutral position and keep your body stationary from hips to shoulders throughout the set. Contract your back muscles as the bar touches your chest and your elbows move behind you. Release the weight slowly and with control (again, don't allow your torso to move) until your arms are fully extended; you should feel a stretch in your back muscles.

**FIFTY SAYS** | "To get the most from this move, I like to think about pulling the weight with my elbows instead of with my hands. That helps me recruit the big muscles of my back."

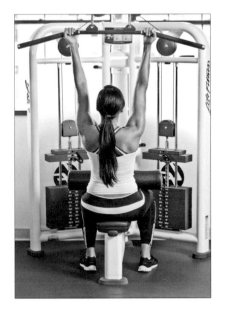

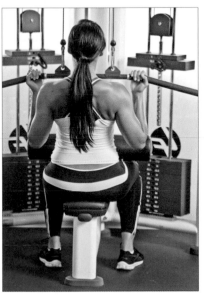

**BASIC MOVE**

# Biceps Curl

**SPECIAL FEATURES** | Dumbbell, 90-degree angle

**TARGET** | Biceps

**PURPOSE** | To work the biceps muscles.

**GET READY** | Set the back support of a bench so that it's nearly vertical. Sit with your back against the upright pad and hold a pair of dumbbells at your sides with your palms facing forward.

**GO** | Curl both weights up close to your shoulders. Keep your upper arms in the same position, perpendicular to the ground, throughout the set. Squeeze both biceps. Lower the dumbbells with control, feeling a stretch in your biceps, until your arms have returned to the starting position.

**FIFTY SAYS** | "When you hold your upper arms still throughout the set, you can't perform as many reps or use as much weight, but you get much better biceps benefits. That really helps you target them."

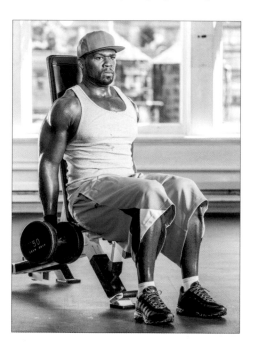 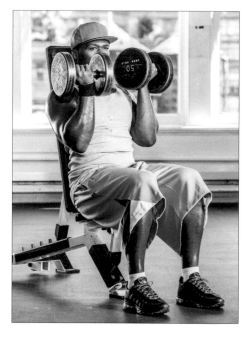

# Rear Delt Raise

**SPECIAL FEATURES** | Dumbbell, prone, 30-degree angle, neutral grip

**TARGET** | Rear delts

**PURPOSE** | To isolate the rear head of your delts. This muscle is difficult for many to isolate and develop—hence the inclusion of this move.

**GET READY** | Lie facedown on a 30 degree incline bench with your chest supported by the pad and your chin extending beyond the top of the bench. Hold a dumbbell in each hand, letting them hang at your sides, arms straight and palms facing each other.

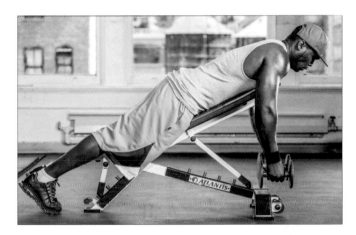

**GO** | Maintaining only a slight bend at your elbows throughout the entire set, raise the weights out to the sides until your arms form a straight line across your shoulder girdle. Contract the muscles between your shoulder joints and back, but avoid shrugging into the move (using your traps), as this undercuts the work that the rear delts perform. Slowly lower the weights to the starting position, emphasizing a stretch in your rear delts.

**FIFTY SAYS** | "You can also perform this move on a T-bar row bench. Some people may find that a more comfortable way to hit this tricky little muscle."

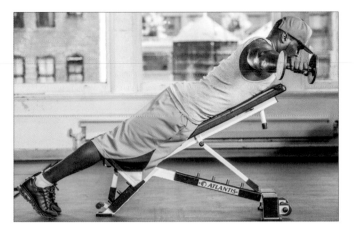

**BASIC MOVE**

# Plank

**SPECIAL FEATURES** | Standard

**TARGET** | Abs, core

**PURPOSE** | To strengthen your core, giving it muscular endurance to better support other weight-training moves.

**GET READY** | Lie facedown on a mat, resting on your forearms with your palms flat on the floor and your elbows directly under your shoulders.

**GO** | Push your hips off the floor by contracting your core muscles, raising up onto your toes. Keep your back flat, forming a straight line from head to heels. Hold this position as long as you can with proper form. When your form begins to fail, lower to the ground and rest for a few seconds. Perform as many reps as it takes to achieve the total time for the set.

**FIFTY SAYS** | "These really make you sweat, but the strength benefits help you excel at other exercises."

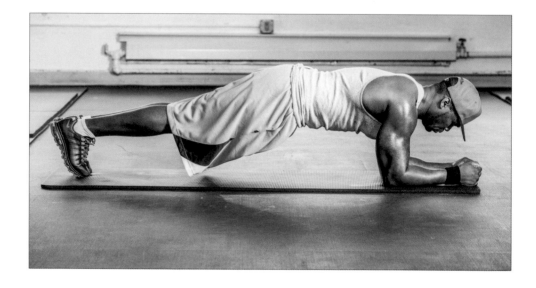

# Phase 2: Weeks 3–6

The biggest difference here is that there are now two alternating resistance-training workouts: Strength 2-A and Strength 2-B.

| Week | Monday | Tuesday | Wednesday | Thursday | Friday | Saturday | Sunday |
|------|--------|---------|-----------|----------|--------|----------|--------|
| #3 | Strength 2-A | EST 2 | Strength 2-B | EST 2 | Strength 2-A | Off | Off |
| #4 | Strength 2-B | EST 2 | Strength 2-A | EST 2 | Strength 2-B | Off | Off |
| #5 | Strength 2-A | EST 2 | Strength 2-B | EST 2 | Strength 2-A | Off | Off |
| #6 | Strength 2-B | EST 2 | Strength 2-A | EST 2 | Strength 2-B | Off | Off |

EST = Energy System Training

## EST 2

During these 4 weeks, each session should begin and end with a leisurely paced 3 to 5 minutes on a treadmill or other cardio apparatus. These are your warm-up and cool-down.

**Week 3**: You're going to do 5 intervals, although you need to go hard for only 2 minutes at a time before backing off to a slower pace for a minute.

**Week 4**: Same drill, only I want you to squeeze out 6 intervals for me.

**Week 5**: Go back to 5 intervals, but up your speed/intensity a bit.

**Week 6**: Same drill, only I want you to squeeze out 6 intervals for me.

## STRENGTH 2-A

### Dynamic Warm-Up/Flexiblity

| Exercise | Sets | Reps | Load | Tempo | Rest | Intensity |
|---|---|---|---|---|---|---|
| Spine Twist | 1 | 5/side | Body-weight | Moderate | None | Low |
| Kneeling Hip Opener | 1 | 5 | Body-weight | Moderate | None | Low |
| Twisting Lunge Stretch | 1 | 5/side | Body-weight | Moderate | None | Low |
| Side Squat | 1 | 5/side | Body-weight | Moderate | None | Low |

### Activation Drills

| Drill | Sets | Reps | Load | Tempo[1] | Rest | Intensity |
|---|---|---|---|---|---|---|
| Lateral Walk | 1 | 10–12/side | Body-weight | 2011 | None | Low |
| Standing W-Raise | 1 | 10 | Body-weight | 2011 | None | Low |

### Strength Training

| Exercise | Sets[2] | Reps | Load[3] | Tempo[1] | Rest (secs) | Intensity |
|---|---|---|---|---|---|---|
| A1. Squat | 3 | 10–12 | TBD | 3010 | ** | Moderate |
| A2. Bench Press | 3 | 10–12 | TBD | 3010 | ** | Moderate |
| B1. Kettlebell Swing | 3 | 10–12 | TBD | Fast | ** | Moderate |
| B2. Dumbbell Row | 3 | 10–12/side | TBD | 3010 | ** | Moderate |
| C1. Push-Up | 3 | To failure | Body-weight | 2010 | ** | Moderate |
| C2. Face Pull | 3 | 10–12 | TBD | 2011 | ** | Moderate |
| D1. Ball Rollout | 3 | 30 seconds | Body-weight | 2020 | 60, 45 | Moderate |

[1] "Tempo" refers to the speed of movement. For example, 3-1-1-0 means: 3 seconds lowering the weight; 1 second pause in the lengthened position; 1 second to raise the weight; no pause ("0") in the contracted position.

[2] When you see exercises preceded by the same letter, complete those sets before moving on to the next pairing. For example, do a set of squats (A1), rest 60 seconds, do a set of bench presses (A2), rest 60 seconds, and then do another set of squats. Only after finishing all 3 sets of each of these exercises do you proceed to the next pairing (B, in this case). Perform those paired sets in the same fashion.

[3] Choose a weight that causes you to fail in the rep range.

** Week 3: Rest 60 seconds between exercise pairings. Week 4: Rest 45 seconds after A1, B1, and C1, and 60 seconds after A2, B2, and C2. Week 5: Rest 30 seconds after A1, B1, and C1, and 60 seconds after A2, B2, and C2. Week 6: Rest 15 seconds after A1, B1, and C1, and 60 seconds after A2, B2, and C2.

**Flexibility training:** Perform immediately post-workout. See Chapter 6, page 61, for details.

**Foam rolling:** Perform immediately after stretching. See Chapter 6, page 72, for details.

## DYNAMIC WARM-UP/FLEXIBILITY
### BASIC MOVE
# Spine Twist (on all fours)

**PURPOSE** | To start your workout by warming up your core as well as preparing your shoulder joints for the work to come.

**GET READY** | On all fours, place your hands directly below your shoulders, and your knees under your hips. With your toes on the ground, take your right hand and place it behind your head.

**GO** | Keep your lower back still and drive your right elbow up toward the ceiling, opening your shoulder joint. You may feel some tightness as you open your chest. Pause for a second at the top, then drive your right elbow down toward elbow. Go as far as you can without allowing your lower back to move. Repeat until you've completed all reps on one side, then switch sides.

**FIFTY SAYS** | "An amazing warm-up move and a great stretch. Sometimes I do this one when I'm tight even if I'm not able to work out."

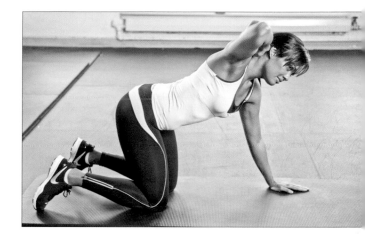

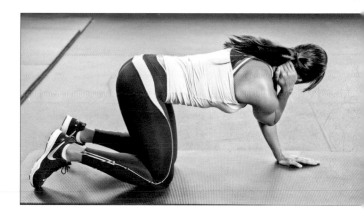

# Kneeling Hip Opener

**PURPOSE** | To open your hips and groin.

**GET READY** | Get down on your hands and knees, placing your hands underneath your shoulders. Your knees should be placed a couple inches wider than your hips, but your feet should be closer together than that.

**GO** | Press your hips back toward your heels, feeling a stretch in your groin. Hold that for a couple seconds and then press your hips forward, returning to the start position.

**FIFTY SAYS** | "This is a classic move, and I strongly recommend you do it frequently if you have problems with tightness in your hips or groin."

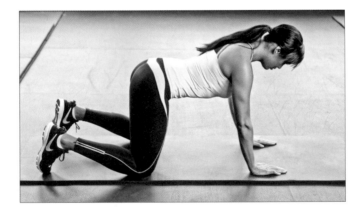

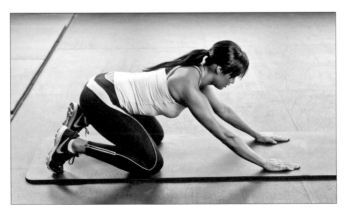

# Twisting Lunge Stretch

**PURPOSE** | To further open your shoulders and groin, and to warm up your core.

**GET READY** | Start by standing tall with feet hip-width apart and chest up and open.

**GO** | Lunge forward with your right leg, straightening your back leg. Place your left hand firmly on the ground, and drive the elbow of your right arm down to your front instep. Feel the stretch in your groin. Next, while keeping your left hand on the ground, and your back leg straight, rotate your right arm up to the ceiling so that your arms form a straight line. Hold that position for a second or 2, then rotate back down to the lunge position. Press back through your front foot, returning to your starting position. Alternate, repeating for the prescribed number of repetitions on each side.

**FIFTY SAYS** | "This may be a warm-up move, but you're gonna feel it working."

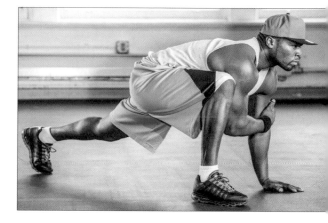

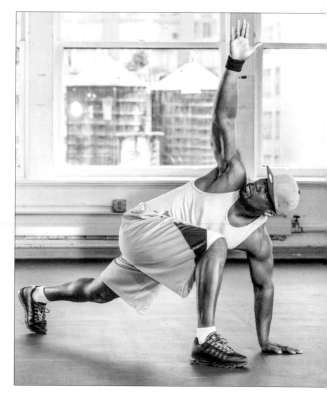

## BASIC MOVE
# Side Squat

**PURPOSE** | To open your groin and warm up your hips, preparing you for the first move in the "Activation Drills" part of the workout, the Lateral Walk (with resistance).

**GET READY** | Stand with your feet about twice as wide as your shoulders.

**GO** | While keeping your right leg straight, lower your hips and push them back a bit to the left. Bend your left knee, keeping your weight on your left heel. Keep both feet fully in contact with the floor, facing forward. Pause for a second at the bottom of the stretch, then return to the starting position by pushing through your left foot. Perform all reps for that side, then perform the same number on the other.

**FIFTY SAYS** | "This stretch is a great prep for the mini-band move that comes next. My stretches, activation drills, and strength moves are all sequenced to get the most from your body in every workout, regardless of your fitness level."

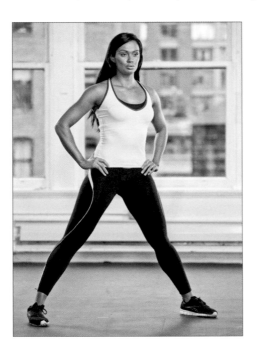 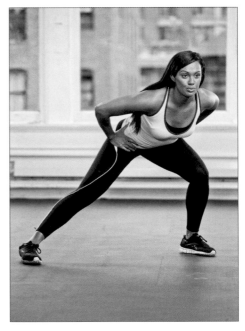

## ACTIVATION DRILLS
### BASIC MOVE
# Lateral Walk (with resistance)

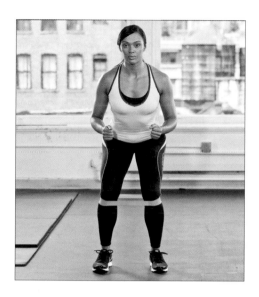 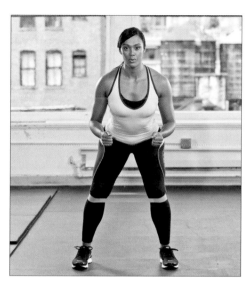

**PURPOSE** | To stretch your hips and add resistance after they've been warmed up.

**GET READY** | Place a mini-band around your legs, just above the knees. Stand with your knees slightly bent and shoulder-width apart, activating the tension in the band.

**GO** | Step to the right and push into the ground with your left foot, keeping your knees bent. As you move your right leg, focus on leading with your knee rather than your foot, keeping tension on the band to recruit the desired muscles. Place your right foot on the ground, stretching the band. Move your left leg laterally toward your right so that there is the same amount of tension as there was at the start of the movement. Continue moving in that direction for the desired number of reps, then do the same in the opposite direction.

**FIFTY SAYS** | "You could turn this activation move into a tough lower-body workout by performing enough reps."

**BASIC MOVE**

# Standing W-Raise

**PURPOSE** | To open your shoulders while retracting your scapula, loosening the upper-back muscles for better range of motion in your shoulders.

**GET READY** | Place your feet shoulder-width apart, bending at your hips until your upper body makes a 45-degree angle with the floor. You can bend slightly at the knees to make the position more comfortable. Keep your upper arms at your sides, with your elbows bent 90 degrees.

**GO** | Keeping your shoulder blades back and down, raise your arms until they form a "W." Your thumbs should be pointed toward each other at the top of the move. Return to the start position and complete the target number of reps.

**FIFTY SAYS** | "As with the Y stretch, this W stretch is a great way to open your shoulders. If you have trouble with tightness in your shoulders, then you can perform these activation moves even when you're not working out."

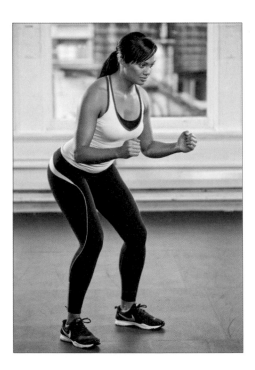 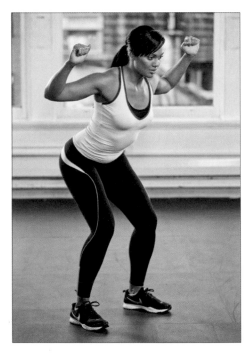

## STRENGTH TRAINING

**BASIC MOVE**

# Squat

**SPECIAL FEATURES** | Kettlebell or dumbbell

**TARGET** | Quads, glutes, hamstrings, core

**PURPOSE** | To train your body as a squat would while preparing you for kettlebell swings in the next superset.

**GET READY** | Hold a kettlebell with both hands at your upper chest, elbows pointing down. Stand tall with your feet slightly wider than your hips. Tighten your back and core muscles to make sure the weight stays close to your body throughout the set.

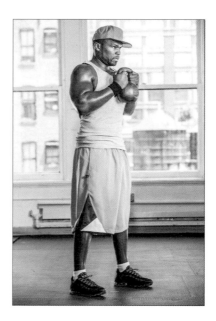

**GO** | Drop your hips back and down, continuing to descend into a full squat position with your body weight on your heels and your thighs below parallel. Go as deep into the squat as you can while maintaining a flat back with your chest up. Allow the kettlebell to counterbalance the backward shift of your body weight as you lower. Drive through your feet to reverse the motion until you return to standing.

**FIFTY SAYS** | "You can tell these squats are working when you start having trouble holding the weight close to your chest."

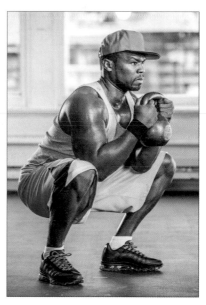

**BASIC MOVE**

# Bench Press

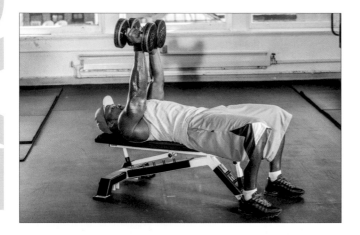

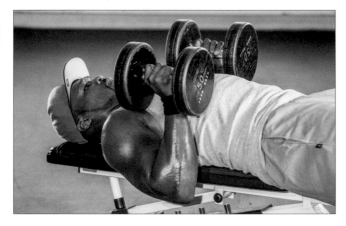

**SPECIAL FEATURES** | Flat bench, dumbbells, neutral grip

**TARGET** | Chest muscles

**PURPOSE** | To work your muscles from a variety of angles using different equipment and hand positions. This is just one variation that helps you achieve complete pectoral development.

**GET READY** | Lie on a flat bench and plant your feet on the floor. Hold a dumbbell in each hand at the side of your pecs, with your palms facing each other and your arms making about a 45-degree angle with your torso. Fully extend your arms toward the ceiling.

**GO** | Hold your shoulders down, chest up and shoulder blades together as you lower the dumbbells until they are directly above your shoulders, palms still facing each other. Lower the weights with control, stretching your pecs as you pull the weights down. Make sure your forearms are perpendicular to the ground throughout the entire set, with your elbows directly under the dumbbells. Press the dumbbells back up to complete the rep.

**FIFTY SAYS** | "This bench press variation lets me take the weights deeper than I can with a barbell, stretching my pecs more. I can really feel the stretch and flex in the portion of the muscle at the separation."

# Kettlebell Swing

**SPECIAL FEATURES** | Two-handed

**TARGET** | Legs, glutes, core

**PURPOSE** | To acclimate your body to yet another type of muscular stimulation by incorporating an explosive move that comes from your legs and hips.

**GET READY** | Stand with your legs shoulder-width apart, holding a kettlebell with both hands. Hold a bend at your knees, allowing the kettlebell to hang between your legs.

**GO** | Bend at the hips, keeping your back flat and shoulders down, and allow the kettlebell to swing between your legs. Your upper body should be close to parallel to the ground. Reverse the motion of the kettlebell by forcefully contracting your hamstrings and glutes to propel the kettlebell forward. Keep your arms straight. You should not be using them to move the weight. All the force comes from the hips. As the kettlebell moves forward, keep your back tight, shoulders down, and chest up. As the weight starts to slow down and reverse direction, let the kettlebell travel back between your legs as you bend at the hips once again.

**FIFTY SAYS** | "Form is crucial to get the most from this move. Stop when you can no longer perform a rep with good form."

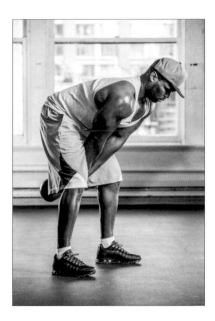

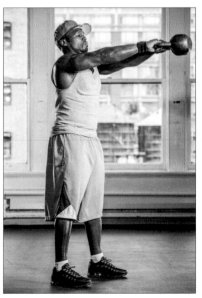

BASIC MOVE

## BASIC MOVE
# Dumbbell Row

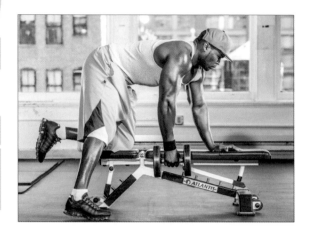

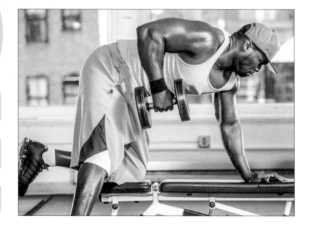

**SPECIAL FEATURES** | Bent over, supported, neutral grip

**TARGET** | Lats

**PURPOSE** | To allow for a deeper contraction than you'd get from many bilateral moves: This move allows you to pull the weight farther than many bilateral moves do because your torso doesn't stop the movement.

**GET READY** | Place one hand and the same-side knee on a flat bench. Hold your back flat and parallel to the floor. Place your other foot beside the bench for support. Grasp a dumbbell with your free hand, keeping your arm straight and your palm facing in toward the bench.

**GO** | Start by bending your arm and pulling the weight to the side of your torso, keeping your back flat and parallel to the floor. Prevent your shoulder joint from dropping or raising throughout the rep. At the top of the movement, contract the muscles in your back and hold for a second. Slowly lower the dumbbell to the start position, feeling a stretch in your lats, until your arm is fully extended.

**FIFTY SAYS** | "You can move a lot more weight if you don't keep this move strict, but if you want to develop size and detail in your back, then make sure your form is spot-on."

# Push-Up

See page 95 for description.

# Face Pull

**SPECIAL FEATURES** | Standing, offset, rope, high, external rotation

**TARGET** | Lats, small muscles of upper back

**PURPOSE** | This move focuses on the upper region of the back, helping to add size and detail to the smaller muscles of the back as well as the upper portion of your lats.

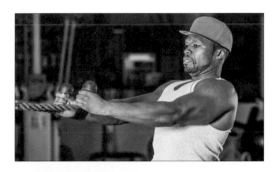

**GET READY** | Attach a rope handle to a cable station and set the pulley to about shoulder height. Grab the rope with straight arms with your knuckles pointing away from you and your thumbs turned in toward your body. Take a couple of steps away from the pulley station with a split stance, one foot behind your body. You should feel tension on the rope. Make sure that your chest is up, shoulders down, and core braced.

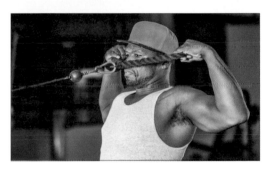

**GO** | Initiate the movement by retracting your shoulder blades, flaring your elbows out, and pulling the rope toward your face. Spread the rope as you pull, maintaining proper posture. Hold the rope in your hands near your ears for a second, feeling a contraction in your back. Slowly allow the weight to return to the start position, focusing on a stretch in your back.

**FIFTY SAYS** | "I like to switch foot positions for each set during this exercise to make sure that I work both sides equally."

# Ball Rollout

**SPECIAL FEATURES** | Palms together

**TARGET** | Abs, serratus

**PURPOSE** | This exercise works many of the muscles of your core through a challenging range of motion.

**GET READY** | Place your hands on an exercise ball with your palms placed together. Start with a slight bend at your hips and shoulders. Brace your core before you begin the movement.

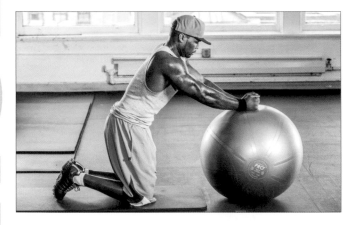

**GO** | Slowly roll the ball forward, straightening your arms and extending your hips. The farther you extend, the more challenging it becomes. Return to the starting position by contracting your abs and rolling the ball back toward your knees. Make sure your back is flat and your core is tight throughout the set.

**FIFTY SAYS** | "I love this move because you can make it so intense by pushing the ball and your limits."

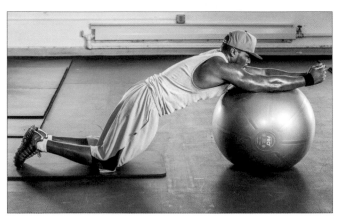

# STRENGTH 2-B

## Dynamic Warm-Up/Flexibility

| Exercise | Sets | Reps | Load | Tempo | Rest | Intensity |
|---|---|---|---|---|---|---|
| Spine Twist | 1 | 5/side | Body-weight | Moderate | None | Low |
| Kneeling Hip Opener | 1 | 5 | Body-weight | Moderate | None | Low |
| Twisting Lunge Stretch | 1 | 5/side | Body-weight | Moderate | None | Low |
| Side Squat | 1 | 5/side | Body-weight | Moderate | None | Low |

## Activation Drills

| Drill | Sets | Reps | Load | Tempo[1] | Rest | Intensity |
|---|---|---|---|---|---|---|
| Lateral Walk | 1 | 10–12/side | Body-weight | 2011 | None | Low |
| Standing W-Raise | 1 | 10 | Body-weight | 2011 | None | Low |

## Strength Training

| Exercise | Sets[2] | Reps | Load[3] | Tempo[1] | Rest (secs) | Intensity |
|---|---|---|---|---|---|---|
| A1. Reverse Lunge | 3 | 10–12/side | TBD | 2010 | ** | Moderate |
| A2. Bench Press | 3 | 10–12 | TBD | 2010 | ** | Moderate |
| B1. Leg Curl | 3 | 10–12 | TBD | 3010 | ** | Moderate |
| B2. Dumbbell Row | 3 | 10–12/side | TBD | 2011 | ** | Moderate |
| C1. Push-Up | 3 | To failure | Body-weight | 2010 | ** | Moderate |
| C2. Biceps Curl | 3 | 8–10 | TBD | 3010 | ** | Moderate |
| D1. Side Plank | 3 | 45 seconds/side | Body-weight | Hold | 60, 45 | Moderate |

[1] "Tempo" refers to the speed of movement. For example, 3-1-1-0 means: 3 seconds lowering the weight; 1 second pause in the lengthened position; 1 second to raise the weight; no pause ("0") in the contracted position.

[2] When you see exercises preceded by the same letter, complete those sets before moving on to the next pairing. For example, do a set of lunges (A1), rest 60 seconds, do a set of bench presses (A2), rest 60 seconds, and then do another set of lunges. Only after finishing all 3 sets for each of those exercises do you proceed to the next pairing (B, in this case). Perform those paired sets in the same fashion.

[3] Choose a weight that causes you to fail in the rep range.

** Week 3: Rest 60 seconds between exercise pairings. Week 4: Rest 45 seconds after A1, B1, and C1, and 60 seconds after A2, B2, and C2. Week 5: Rest 30 seconds after A1, B1, and C1, and 60 seconds after A2, B2, and C2. Week 6: Rest 15 seconds after A1, B1, and C1, and 45 seconds after A2, B2, and C2.

**Flexibility training:** Perform immediately post-workout. See Chapter 6, page 61, for details.

**Foam rolling:** Perform immediately after stretching. See Chapter 6, page 72, for details.

## STRENGTH TRAINING

**BASIC MOVE**

# Reverse Lunge

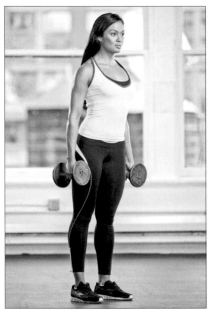

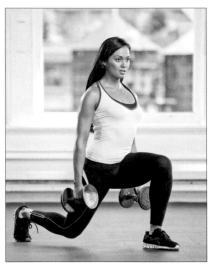

**SPECIAL FEATURES** | Dumbbells

**TARGET** | Hamstrings, glutes, quads, core

**PURPOSE** | This move recruits all the major muscles of your legs while also challenging your core to maintain your balance throughout the set.

**GET READY** | Hold a dumbbell in each hand at your side, palms facing in. Place your feet hip-width apart and pull your chest up.

**GO** | Step one leg back 2 to 3 feet. Squeeze your glutes as your back foot hits the ground, then lower into a lunge position. Bend your front leg as you do this, keeping your back knee from hitting the floor. Make certain that your front knee doesn't travel past your toes, keeping your lower leg nearly perpendicular to the ground. Keep your hips and core engaged throughout. To return to the start position, drive through your front leg while maintaining your upright posture until you return to your upright position. Complete all reps for one leg, then perform the same number on the other side.

**FIFTY SAYS** | "I think these are even more challenging than regular lunges. They really work your balance and core."

# Bench Press

**SPECIAL FEATURES** | Dumbbell, incline, neutral grip

**TARGET** | Upper pecs

**PURPOSE** | This move allows a deep stretch in your pecs, while the angle promotes growth in the upper chest.

**GET READY** | Set a bench at a 30-degree incline and place the dumbbells on your knees after you sit down. Lie back on the bench and use your legs to help get the dumbbells to their start position with your arms extended and the dumbbells over your shoulders.

**GO** | Lower the dumbbells with control, holding your upper arms at 45 degrees from your body. Lower the weights until your elbows are slightly below shoulder level. Feel the stretch in your pecs at the bottom of the move. Keeping your chest up and shoulders back, press the dumbbells up until your arms are fully extended. Emphasize the contraction in your pectorals.

**FIFTY SAYS** | "I like to use different angles to hit my muscle groups in different ways. This type of bench press really pumps my upper chest."

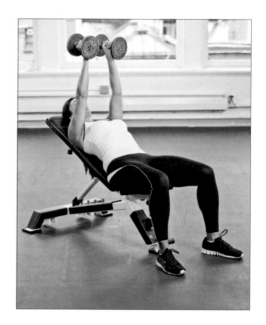

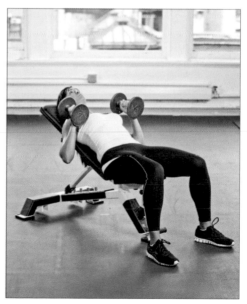

## BASIC MOVE
# Leg Curl

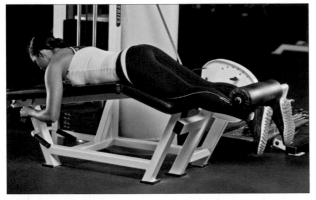

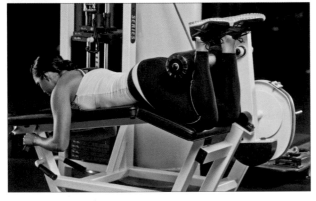

**SPECIAL FEATURES** | Prone, machine

**TARGET** | Hamstrings

**PURPOSE** | This move isolates the hamstrings, which are sometimes undertrained during whole-leg moves such as squats.

**GET READY** | Lie facedown on a prone leg curl machine with the leg pad adjusted so that it rests on your lower calves. Your knees should be in line with the machine's joint of rotation. Your legs should be fully extended at the start. Flex your feet (pull your toes toward your shins) and hold them in that position throughout the set to better target the hamstrings.

**GO** | Keeping your back flat, core tight, and head down, begin to curl your lower legs toward your glutes. Think about getting your heels to your butt as you curl your lower legs. Hold a contraction in your hamstrings for a second at the top of the movement, then return the weight to the start, slowly letting your heels move away from your glutes, keeping your glutes and hamstrings contracted the entire time. Lower the weight until your legs are fully extended and you feel a stretch in your hamstrings.

**FIFTY SAYS** | "Keep the motion smooth throughout—don't jerk the weight or round your lower back. That risks injury and undercuts the work that you want your hamstrings to perform."

# Dumbbell Row

**SPECIAL FEATURES** | Bent over, supported, pronated grip, elbow extended

**TARGET** | Lats, smaller muscles of the upper back

**PURPOSE** | Dumbbell rows allow for a greater range of motion and deeper contraction than many two-handed back moves such as pull-downs and barbell rows.

**GET READY** | Place one hand and your same-side knee on a flat bench. Hold your back flat and close to parallel to the floor. Place your other foot next to the bench for support. With your free hand, grab a dumbbell and keep your arm straight, palm facing toward the knee of the foot that's on the floor. Hold your shoulders down and back throughout the set

**GO** | Initiate the movement by bending your arm and pulling the weight away from your torso, keeping that shoulder down, your back flat and parallel to the floor. Your elbow should be rotated out so that your upper arm is perpendicular to your torso

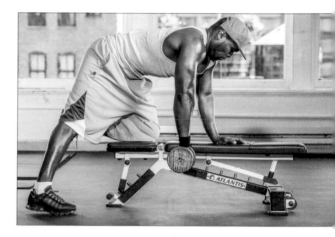

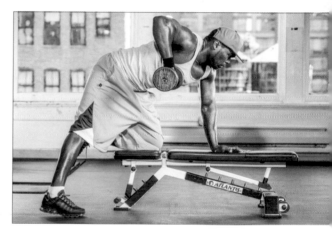

at the top of the movement. Contract the muscles of your upper back and hold for a second. Then slowly lower the dumbbell to the start position, feeling a stretch in those same back muscles. Complete reps for both arms.

**FIFTY SAYS** | "The pronated grip makes this type of dumbbell row more challenging than the neutral-grip version. I use a little less weight for these."

## BASIC MOVE
# Push-Up

See page 95 for description.

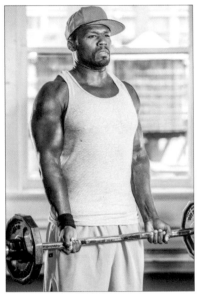

## BASIC MOVE
# Biceps Curl

**SPECIAL FEATURES** | EZ-curl bar

**TARGET** | Works your biceps bilaterally

**PURPOSE** | The hand position is about the width of your elbows.

**GET READY** | Grab an EZ-curl bar with a medium, palms-up grip, hands shoulder-width. Stand tall with your feet slightly wider than your hips. Keep your chest up and shoulders down.

**GO** | Keep your elbows at your sides, in line with your body, and curl the weight toward your shoulders by contracting your biceps. Do not swing the weight or lean back to complete the lift. Once the weight is at your shoulders, force a deeper contraction into your biceps. Then reverse the motion, letting the weight slowly travel away from your body, controlling the movement with your biceps, returning the weight to the starting position. Keep your upper arms still throughout the set.

**FIFTY SAYS** | "This is a terrific biceps pumper. Because you're training both arms at the same time, you work your biceps continuously during the set, really driving blood into the muscles."

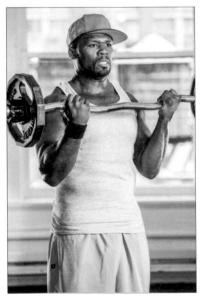

# Side Plank

**SPECIAL FEATURES** | Standard

**TARGET** | Core, shoulders, whole body

**PURPOSE** | This move recruits whole-body muscular endurance, especially targeting your abs, stabilizer muscles, and shoulders, encouraging overall conditioning and definition.

**GET READY** | Lean on your side with your elbow under your shoulder, supporting some of your body weight. With straight legs, stack your feet on top of each other so only the lower one contacts the ground.

**GO** | Raise your body off the ground by pressing your elbow into the ground, squeezing your glutes and contracting your core. Your elbow should be directly under your shoulder, and your body should form a straight line from your head to your feet. Hold for as long as you can while keeping good form. Rest for a few seconds if necessary, then perform as many reps as needed to achieve the total working time of the set. Turn onto the other side and complete all reps on that side as well.

**FIFTY SAYS** | "This is another move that's more difficult than it looks. As you get accustomed to performing it, you'll also notice that your muscular endurance is increasing for other weight-training exercises."

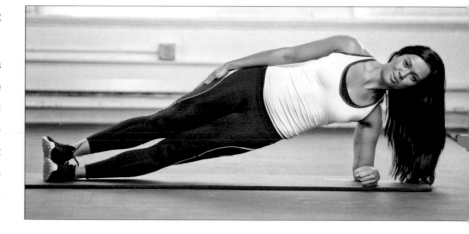

# 8

# Formula 50, the Meal Plan

I F YOU'RE ONE OF THOSE PEOPLE WHO THINK DIET IS JUST one letter removed from "die," you're in for a big surprise when you check out the meal plans for Formula 50. Based on my own food preferences and diet philosophy, they were designed for you by Stephanie M. C. Wilson, MS, RD, CISSN, LDN, Head of Nutrition at IMG Academies. Formerly, she served as Sports Nutrition Consultant for the University of South Florida athletic department. Stephanie's athletic background includes having been a gymnast and runner. She earned the American Dietetic Association Outstanding Dietetic Intern of the Year Award in 2009.

There are two sets of meal plans, one for men, using a 185-pounder as an example; and one for women, using a

135-pounder as an example. If you weigh more or less than those amounts, adjust your caloric intake accordingly while keeping the protein-carb-fat allocation the same. Use percentages. For example, if you're a dude who weighs 10 percent more than 185 pounds, bump your total calories up by 10 percent, dividing them more or less equally among your meals.

The 6 weeks are covered by three weekly meal plans, so I'm giving twenty-one meals for the guys and another twenty-one for the ladies. The first seven cover Weeks 1–2, the next seven cover Weeks 3–4, and the final seven cover Weeks 5–6. So each new week's menu is followed by one repeat week. The meals themselves are so diverse that boredom won't set in over a mere 14 days. In fact, the repetition should make it a little easier for you to manage your food shopping and preparation.

If you go on to do the advanced phase after this first phase, go through the meal plans in sequence again. They'll work equally well.

Finally, these meal plans are examples, not mandatory, set-in-stone, follow-this-exactly-or-else edicts. If you can follow them more or less to the T, great; if you can't, replace those items you can't make or acquire with similar items. Swapping beef for chicken or fish won't make a difference; swapping an orange for a cinnamon roll will make a difference, and a huge one if you do it often. Learn to read labels, learn to cook, and learn to use good judgment when it comes to food. All will hold you in good stead for the duration of Formula 50 and beyond.

## Men's (185 pounds) Meal Plan, Weeks 1–2

### Day 1

**BREAKFAST**
24 raw almonds
*Protein-Packed Oatmeal*
½ cup oatmeal
1 scoop vanilla whey protein
¼ cup blueberries

**LUNCH**
*Chicken Sandwich*
6 ounces grilled chicken
2 slices reduced-calorie wheat bread
2 tbsp low-calorie BBQ sauce

1½ cups steamed broccoli, chopped,
    with 1 tbsp olive oil

**DINNER**
5 ounces sirloin
1 large sweet potato (3 x 6 inches)
1 cup steamed green beans, with
    1 tbsp olive oil

**SNACK**

*Berry-Nut Yogurt*

6 ounces nonfat plain Greek
   yogurt

2 cups strawberries

6 walnuts, halved

non-calorie sweetener

**POST-WORKOUT**

16 ounces Gatorade with 1½ scoops
   whey protein

## Day 2

**BREAKFAST**

2 high-fiber waffles with calorie-free
   syrup and butter spray

½ cup egg whites + 1 egg, scrambled,
   with ¼ cup shredded cheese (regular)

1 cup fresh mixed fruit

**LUNCH**

6 ounces blackened shrimp

¾ cup brown rice

¼ cup black beans

½ cup steamed spinach with 2 tbsp
   olive oil

**DINNER**

*Fish Tacos*

6 ounces grilled chili-seasoned tilapia

3 small corn tortillas (4½ inches)

2 cups romaine lettuce

¼ avocado, sliced

**SNACK**

*Blended Smoothie*

1 scoop whey protein

8 ounces 1% milk

ice

2 cups strawberries

1 small banana (6–7 inches)

**POST-WORKOUT**

16 ounces Gatorade with 1½ scoops
   whey protein

## Day 3

**BREAKFAST**

*Apple-Nut Oatmeal*

½ cup oatmeal

1 cup sliced apples

cinnamon and non-calorie sweetener

1 scoop vanilla whey protein

14 walnuts, halved

**LUNCH**

*Cheeseburger*

5 ounces grilled 96% lean ground
   beef

2 slices reduced-calorie wheat bread

2 tbsp ketchup

1-ounce slice American cheese

2 cups sliced zucchini

### DINNER

6 ounces lemon pepper chicken

1 cup whole-grain pasta

2 cups sliced summer squash

### SNACK

*Berry-Nut Yogurt*

8 ounces nonfat plain Greek yogurt

2 cups blueberries

14 walnuts, halved

non-calorie sweetener

### POST-WORKOUT

16 ounces Gatorade with 1½ scoops
   whey protein

## Day 4

### BREAKFAST

*Breakfast Sandwich*

3 slices Canadian bacon

1 egg

1 whole-wheat English muffin

1 ounce shredded American cheese
   (regular)

1 small banana (6–7 inches)

### LUNCH

*Chicken Pita*

6 ounces buffalo deli nonfat chicken

1 slice medium tomato (¼-inch thick)

½ cup alfalfa sprouts

2 tbsp light ranch dressing

1 small whole-wheat pita

### DINNER

*Steak Salad*

5 ounces black pepper sirloin

3 cups romaine lettuce

½ cup cucumber slices

½ cup fresh yellow corn

¼ cup black beans

2 tbsp light creamy Parmesan ranch
   dressing

### SNACK

14 raw almonds

*Blended Smoothie*

8 ounces of 1% milk

ice

2 cups mixed berries

### POST-WORKOUT

16 ounces Gatorade with 1½ scoops whey
   protein

## Day 5

### BREAKFAST

*Egg Pita*

1 egg and ¾ cup egg substitute

1 ounce shredded low-fat cheddar cheese

1 whole-wheat pita

¼ cup mushrooms, cooked

¼ cup cooked spinach with 2 tsp olive oil

1 cup sugar-free kiwi strawberry drink
   mix

1 plum

LUNCH

*Chicken Wrap*

1 low-carb, low-fat, high-fiber wrap

5 ounces chicken, sliced

2 tbsp fajita seasoning

1 ounce pepper jack cheese (regular)

1 cup mixed chopped green pepper,
onion, red pepper, cooked in 1 tbsp
olive oil

DINNER

5 ounces Jamaican jerk salmon, broiled

¾ cup brown rice

2 cups asparagus

SNACK

24 raw almonds

*Mango Yogurt*

1 cup sliced mangos

8 ounces nonfat pineapple
Greek yogurt

POST-WORKOUT

16 ounces Gatorade with 1½ scoops
whey protein

## Day 6

BREAKFAST

*Chocolate Peanut Butter Oatmeal*

½ cup oatmeal

1 scoop chocolate whey protein

1 tbsp unsweetened cocoa

2 tbsp peanut butter

LUNCH

*Turkey Sandwich*

4 ounces turkey breast

2 slices reduced-calorie wheat bread

2 tbsp mustard

2 ounces Swiss cheese

2 cups mixed steamed carrots, broccoli,
and cauliflower

DINNER

*Kabobs*

6 ounces sirloin

½ cup pineapple chunks

½ cup chopped bell pepper

½ cup chopped onion

½ cup brown rice with 1 tbsp
olive oil

SNACK

6 ounces nonfat plain Greek yogurt
mixed with ranch powdered dip

20 baby carrots

1 ounce low-calorie baked chips with
½ cup salsa

## Day 7

BREAKFAST

*Cheese and Spinach Eggs*

1 cup egg substitute

¼ cup shredded nonfat cheese

1 cup cooked spinach

¼ cup (cooked in water) whole-grain grits

## LUNCH

*Pasta Salad*

1 cup cooked broccoli florets

¼ cup pasta

2 tbsp light Italian dressing

½ cup corn

6 ounces blackened chicken

## DINNER

6 ounces center-cut herb-seasoned pork tenderloin

1 cup steamed green beans with 2 tbsp olive oil

½ baked potato

## SNACK

1 whole-wheat mini bagel with 2 tbsp low-fat cream cheese

14 raw almonds

## Men's (185 Pounds) Meal Plan, Weeks 3–4

### Day 1

**BREAKFAST**

7 raw almonds

2 blueberry high-fiber waffles with butter spray and calorie-free syrup

*Blended Smoothie*

¼ cup frozen blueberries

1 scoop whey protein

ice and water

1 cup halved fresh strawberries

## LUNCH

*Chef Salad*

¾ cup diced extra-lean ham

¼ cup shredded nonfat cheddar cheese

3 cups romaine lettuce

1 large, hard-boiled egg

balsamic vinegar + 2 tbsp light ranch dressing

2 slices reduced-calorie wheat toast with butter spray

1 medium apple, sliced

## DINNER

5 ounces blackened salmon

1 cup couscous

20 small asparagus spears, steamed, with 1 tbsp olive oil

## SNACK

*Turkey Wrap*

1 multi-grain, high-fiber, low-calorie wrap

3 ounces roasted turkey breast (low sodium)

7 raw walnuts

## POST-WORKOUT

16 ounces Gatorade with 1½ scoops whey protein

## Day 2

**BREAKFAST**

*Egg Wrap*

1 multi-grain, high-fiber,
   low-calorie wrap

½ cup egg whites and 1 egg

¼ cup shredded nonfat cheese

⅛ cup steamed spinach

hot sauce

2 cups fresh honeydew/cantaloupe

**LUNCH**

6 ounces basil and garlic shrimp

1 cup spaghetti squash

½ cup chopped red/green pepper

1 cup broccoli, cooked, chopped

2 tbsp olive oil

**DINNER**

5 ounces Jamaican jerk chicken

½ cup brown rice

¼ cup black beans

2 cups green beans, steamed

lemon juice for green beans

1 tbsp olive oil

**SNACK**

20 raw almonds

*Blended Smoothie*

1 scoop whey protein

8 ounces 1% milk

ice

½ cup pineapple chunks (in own juice)

1 cup raspberries

**POST-WORKOUT**

16 ounces Gatorade with 1½ scoops
   whey protein

## Day 3

**BREAKFAST**

10 walnuts, halved

*Vanilla Peach Oatmeal*

½ cup oatmeal

1 cup sliced peach

cinnamon and non-calorie sweetener

1 scoop vanilla whey protein

**LUNCH**

5 ounces beef tenderloin

1 small baked potato

1½ cups mixed roasted zucchini, squash,
   and red pepper with 1 tbsp olive oil

**DINNER**

5 ounces grouper, broiled, topped with
   ⅛ cup mango salsa

¼ cup brown rice

¼ cup black beans

2 cups steamed green/yellow bean mix

**SNACK 1**

*Chocolate-Strawberry Yogurt*

8 ounces nonfat plain Greek yogurt

1 cup halved strawberries

2 tbsp ground flaxseed

1 tbsp unsweetened cocoa

non-calorie sweetener

## SNACK 2

8 ounces nonfat milk

## POST-WORKOUT

16 ounces Gatorade with 1½ scoops
   whey protein

## Day 4

### BREAKFAST

*Breakfast Sandwich*

1 egg and 3¾ cups egg substitute

1 ounce shredded low-fat cheddar
   cheese

1 whole-grain English muffin

¼ cup chopped onion, cooked

¼ cup chopped pepper, cooked

2 tsp olive oil

### LUNCH

*Chicken Salad*

5 ounces grilled chicken, chopped

1 cup cherry tomatoes

¼ cup shredded carrots

½ cup chopped cucumber

3 cups romaine lettuce

2 tbsp light BBQ sauce

2 tbsp light ranch dressing

2 slices reduced-calorie wheat bread
   with butter spray

## DINNER

6 ounces grilled salmon with lemon

1 large sweet potato topped with butter
   spray, cinnamon, and non-calorie
   sweetener

10 pecans, halved

2 cups mixed vegetables (broccoli,
   cauliflower, carrots)

## SNACK

8 ounces 1% milk

1 small banana (6 inches)

13 raw almonds

1 ounce beef jerky

## POST-WORKOUT

16 ounces Gatorade with 1½ scoops
   whey protein

## Day 5

### BREAKFAST

½ cup oatmeal with cinnamon

8 ounces nonfat plain Greek yogurt
   mixed with 1 cup mixed berries and
   non-calorie sweetener

6 raw almonds

### LUNCH

*Sesame Chicken Salad*

5 ounces chicken, sliced

3 cups fresh spinach

1 orange, sliced

½ cup alfalfa sprouts

2 tbsp sesame ginger dressing

2 tsp sesame seeds, toasted

2 slices reduced-calorie wheat bread
with butter spray

### DINNER

**Shrimp Stir-Fry**

6 ounces shrimp

½ cup brown rice

2 cups mixed Asian vegetables

rice vinegar

2 tsp sesame seeds, toasted

ginger/desired spice

2 tbsp olive oil

### SNACK

**Blended Smoothie**

1 scoop vanilla whey protein

8 ounces of 1% milk

ice

1 cup blueberries

### POST-WORKOUT

16 ounces Gatorade with 1½ scoops
whey protein

## Day 6

### BREAKFAST

**Blended Smoothie**

8 ounces 1% milk

ice

1 cup strawberries

1 scoop chocolate whey protein

1 whole-wheat English muffin with
2 tbsp peanut butter

### LUNCH

**Steak Tacos**

4 ounces sirloin

3 small corn tortillas (4½ inches)

2 cups shredded romaine lettuce

¼ cup salsa

¼ cup shredded nonfat mozzarella
cheese

¾ avocado

### DINNER

**Chicken Stir-Fry**

5 ounces chicken

½ cup pineapple chunks

½ cup sliced bell pepper

½ cup brown rice

1 tbsp olive oil

### SNACK 1

6 ounces nonfat plain Greek yogurt
mixed with ranch powdered dip

20 baby carrots

### SNACK 2

¼ cup black bean and corn salsa

1 ounce baked corn chips

## Day 7

**BREAKFAST**

½ cup oatmeal

*Veggie Egg Scramble*

1 cup egg substitute

¼ cup shredded nonfat cheddar cheese

1 cup cooked chopped spinach,
    mushrooms, and tomato

1 tbsp olive oil

**LUNCH**

*Turkey Sandwich*

5 ounces oven roasted turkey

2 slices reduced-calorie wheat bread

1 ounce shredded pepper jack cheese
    (regular)

1 lettuce leaf

1 tomato, sliced

yellow mustard

2 cups steamed broccoli with
    2 tbsp low-fat ranch dressing

1 apple

**DINNER**

5 ounces blackened chicken

5 ounces roasted red potatoes with garlic

20 raw almonds

1 cup steamed green beans

**SNACK**

6 ounces nonfat plain Greek yogurt
    mixed with non-calorie sweetener

1 cup halved fresh strawberries

1 cup mixed melon cubes

## Men's (185 Pounds) Meal Plan, Weeks 5–6

## Day 1

**BREAKFAST**

*Breakfast Sandwich*

3 ounces sliced Canadian bacon

2 hard-boiled eggs

1 whole-wheat English muffin

5 sprays of butter substitute

1 orange (3 inches in diameter)

**LUNCH**

*Buffalo Chicken Sandwich*

5 ounces grilled chicken breast

1 tbsp buffalo sauce marinade

3 cups shredded romaine lettuce

1 ounce part-skim mozzarella cheese

2 slices reduced-calorie wheat bread

1 small apple

**DINNER**

6 ounces shrimp with Jamaican jerk
    spices (as desired)

¾ cup brown rice

2 cups steamed green/yellow bean
    blend

2 tbsp olive oil

**SNACK**

8 ounces nonfat Greek yogurt
(any flavor)
10 raw almonds/walnuts

**POST-WORKOUT**

16 ounces Gatorade with 1½ scoops
whey protein

## Day 2

**BREAKFAST**

7 raw almonds
2 whole-grain, high-fiber waffles
with butter spray and calorie-free
syrup

*Blended Smoothie*
½ extra-small banana
1½ scoops whey protein
ice and water

**LUNCH**

5 ounces grilled flank steak with garlic
1 large sweet potato
1½ cups roasted zucchini and squash
with 1 tbsp olive oil

**DINNER**

5 ounces roast turkey with rosemary,
thyme, basil
2 cups snap green beans and
20 almonds, sauteed in 1 tbsp
olive oil

2 pieces reduced-calorie bread with
1 tbsp butter, whipped

**SNACK**

8 ounces 1% milk with 1 scoop
whey protein
7 walnuts, halved

**POST-WORKOUT**

16 ounces Gatorade with 1½ scoops
whey protein

## Day 3

**BREAKFAST**

*Breakfast Wrap*
1 multi-grain, high-fiber, low-calorie
wrap
1¼ cups egg whites or egg substitute
½ cup chopped fresh mushrooms
¼ cup steamed spinach
pepper-and-olive cooking spray

1½ cups fresh honeydew/cantaloupe

**LUNCH**

5 ounces pork tenderloin with
2 tbsp chipotle pepper marinade
powder

*Dirty Rice*
½ cup brown rice
½ cup chopped jalapeno peppers
½ cup chopped onion

nonfat cooking spray

2 tbsp olive oil

**DINNER**

*Sesame Chicken*

5 ounces boneless, skinless chicken
   breast

2 tbsp Asian ginger marinade

2 cups mixed Asian vegetables

¾ cup couscous

1 tbsp sesame oil

1 tbsp sesame seeds

**SNACK**

2 cups fresh raspberries

20 raw walnuts

1 scoop whey protein mixed in water

**POST-WORKOUT**

16 ounces Gatorade with 1½ scoops
   whey protein

## Day 4

**BREAKFAST**

2 eggs, over easy

1 whole-grain mini bagel with
   2 ounces sliced cheese

*Scrambled Egg Whites*

¼ cup chopped onion

½ cup chopped bell pepper

¾ cup egg whites

nonfat cooking spray

**LUNCH**

*Hawaiian Chicken*

5 ounces chicken tenderloin

3 tbsp low-calorie BBQ sauce

½ cup pineapple chunks

1 cup broccoli florets

½ cup wild rice

**DINNER**

5 ounces blackened shrimp with
   1 tbsp olive oil

1 medium baked potato with
   1 tbsp whipped butter

1 cup cooked spinach with
   2 tsp olive oil

**SNACK**

1 apple

24 raw almonds

6 ounces nonfat Greek yogurt
   (any flavor)

**POST-WORKOUT**

16 ounces Gatorade with 1½ scoops
   whey protein

## Day 5

**BREAKFAST**

1 whole-grain, high-fiber waffle with
   1 tbsp creamy peanut butter

*Blended Smoothie*

1½ scoops chocolate whey protein

1 small banana (6–7 inches)
ice and water

## LUNCH

### *Tequila Lime Tilapia*
1–2 tbsp tequila lime seasoning
5 ounces grilled tilapia

20 small asparagus spears (5 inches
    or less) with 2 tbsp olive oil
½ cup brown rice

## DINNER

### *Beef Tacos*
5 ounces 96% lean ground beef
2 small corn tortillas (4½ inches)
2 cups shredded lettuce
¼ cup salsa
½ cup sliced plum tomatoes
½ cup chopped cucumber

## SNACK
8 ounces nonfat milk with 1 scoop
    whey protein
1 high-fiber granola bar

## POST-WORKOUT
16 ounces Gatorade with 1½ scoops
    whey protein

## Day 6

### BREAKFAST
2 slices reduced-calorie bread with
    1 tbsp whole-fruit spread

2 (1-ounce) slices of Canadian bacon
2 eggs, sunny-side up
1 cup honeydew melon

## LUNCH

### *Cheeseburger*
5 ounces grilled 96% lean ground beef
1 slice nonfat cheese stuffed inside
    burger
1 slice nonfat cheese on top
¼-inch slice tomato
2 slices reduced-calorie wheat bread

### *Salad*
3 cups romaine lettuce
2 tbsp fat-free Caesar dressing

## DINNER
5 ounces herb-crusted salmon
    topped with diced tomato and
    garlic

### *Rice Pilaf*
½ cup brown rice
garlic
¼ cup finely chopped onion
1 tbsp olive oil

## SNACK

### *Blended Smoothie*
8 ounces nonfat milk
½ scoop vanilla whey protein
½ cup mango
1 extra-small banana (less than
    6 inches)

## Day 7

### BREAKFAST

1 whole-wheat English muffin with
   2 tbsp peanut butter

*Blended Smoothie*

1 cup strawberries

½ banana (less than 6 inches)

1 scoop whey protein

ice and water

### LUNCH

5 ounces blackened mahi mahi
   (or other fish)

1 small baked potato topped with
   1 ounce part-skim cheese and
   10 sprays low-calorie butter
   spray

1½ cups mixed vegetables, roasted with
   garlic and 2 tsp olive oil

### DINNER

*Mediterranean-Style Chicken*

5 ounces grilled chicken

1 cup diced, canned tomatoes

1 clove garlic

2 tbsp dried basil

1–2 tbsp diced olives

1 ounce grated Parmesan cheese

*Rice and Peppers*

½ cup yellow rice

1 cup chopped green peppers,
   cooked with rice

1 tbsp olive oil

1 ounce grated Parmesan cheese

### SNACK

¾ cup high-fiber honey-oat cereal with
   8 ounces nonfat milk

## Women's (135 pounds) Meal Plan, Weeks 1–2

## Day 1

### BREAKFAST

12 raw almonds

*Protein-Packed Oatmeal*

½ cup oatmeal

1 scoop vanilla whey protein

¼ cup blueberries

### LUNCH

*Chicken Sandwich*

4 ounces grilled chicken

2 slices reduced-calorie wheat bread

2 tbsp low calorie BBQ Sauce

1 cup steamed broccoli, chopped, with
   2 tsp olive oil

### DINNER

3½ ounces sirloin

½ large sweet potato
   (3 x 6 inches)

2 cups green beans, steamed, with
   2 tsp olive oil

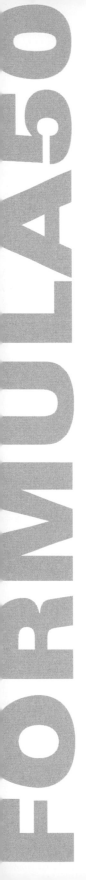

**SNACK**

*Berry-Nut Yogurt*

4 ounces nonfat plain Greek yogurt

1 cup strawberries

14 walnuts, halved

non-calorie sweetener

**POST-WORKOUT**

8 ounces Gatorade with 1 scoop
    whey protein

## Day 2

**BREAKFAST**

1 high-fiber waffle with calorie-free
    syrup and butter spray

⅓ cup egg whites and 1 whole
    egg, scrambled with ¼ cup
    shredded cheddar cheese
    (regular)

1 cup fresh strawberries

**LUNCH**

4 ounces blackened shrimp

½ cup brown rice

¼ cup black beans

1 tbsp olive oil

½ cup steamed spinach

**DINNER**

*Fish Tacos*

4 ounces grilled chili-seasoned
    tilapia

2 small corn tortillas (4½ inches)

2 cups romaine lettuce

¼ avocado, sliced

**SNACK**

*Blended Smoothie*

1 cup strawberries

8 ounces 1% milk

¼ scoop whey protein

**POST-WORKOUT**

8 ounces Gatorade with 1 scoop
    whey protein

## Day 3

**BREAKFAST**

*Vanilla Apple Oatmeal*

½ cup oatmeal

1 cup sliced apples

cinnamon and non-calorie sweetener

1 scoop vanilla whey protein


7 walnuts, halved

**LUNCH**

*Cheeseburger*

4 ounces grilled 96% lean ground
    beef

2 slices reduced-calorie wheat bread

2 tbsp ketchup

1-ounce slice American cheese

1 cup steamed chopped
    zucchini

### DINNER

4 ounces lemon pepper chicken

½ cup whole-grain pasta

2 cups sliced summer squash

### SNACK

*Blueberry-Nut Yogurt*

4 ounces nonfat plain Greek yogurt

1 cup blueberries

14 walnuts, halved

non-calorie sweetener

### POST-WORKOUT

8 ounces Gatorade with 1 scoop
   whey protein

## Day 4

### BREAKFAST

*Breakfast Sandwich*

3 slices Canadian bacon

1 egg

1 whole-wheat English muffin

1 ounce American cheese
   (regular)

1 cup mixed berries (fresh blueberries,
   strawberry halves)

### LUNCH

*Chicken Pita*

4 ounces buffalo deli nonfat
   chicken

1 slice medium tomato (¼-inch
   thick)

½ cup alfalfa sprouts

1 tbsp light ranch dressing

1 small whole-wheat pita

### DINNER

*Steak Salad*

4 ounces black pepper sirloin

3 cups romaine lettuce

½ cup cucumber slices

¼ cup fresh yellow corn

¼ cup black beans

2 tbsp light creamy Parmesan ranch
   dressing

### SNACK

12 raw almonds

*Blended Smoothie*

8 ounces 1% milk

ice

1 cup mixed berries

### POST-WORKOUT

8 ounces Gatorade with 1 scoop
   whey protein

## Day 5

### BREAKFAST

*Breakfast Pita*

1 egg

½ cup egg substitute

½ ounce low-fat cheddar
cheese

1 whole-wheat pita

¼ cup mushrooms, cooked

¼ cup cooked spinach

## LUNCH

*Chicken Wrap*

1 low-carb, low-fat, high-fiber
wrap

3½ ounces chicken, sliced

2 tbsp fajita seasoning

½ ounce pepper jack cheese
(regular)

1 cup mixed chopped green pepper,
onion, red pepper, cooked in
cooking spray, with 2 tsp
olive oil

## DINNER

4 ounces Jamaican jerk spice salmon,
broiled

½ cup brown rice

2 cups asparagus

## SNACK

*Banana-Nut Yogurt*

1 extra-small banana (less than
6 inches)

4 ounces nonfat plain Greek
yogurt

non-calorie sweetener

12 raw almonds

## POST-WORKOUT

8 ounces Gatorade with 1 scoop
whey protein

## Day 6

## BREAKFAST

*Chocolate Peanut Butter Oatmeal*

½ cup oatmeal

1 scoop chocolate whey protein

1 tbsp unsweetened cocoa and non-
calorie sweetener

1 tbsp natural peanut butter

## LUNCH

*Turkey Sandwich*

4 ounces turkey breast

2 slices reduced-calorie wheat bread

2 tbsp mustard

1 cup mixed steamed carrots, broccoli,
and cauliflower

½ apple, quartered

## DINNER

*Kabobs*

4 ounces sirloin

½ cup pineapple chunks

½ cup chopped bell pepper

½ cup chopped onion

½ cup brown rice

2 tbsp olive oil

SNACK

4 ounces nonfat plain Greek yogurt
mixed with ranch powdered dip
20 baby carrots

## Day 7

BREAKFAST

*Breakfast Sandwich*

1 whole-wheat English muffin

½ cup egg substitute

¼ cup shredded nonfat cheese

1 cup cooked spinach

LUNCH

*Chicken Sandwich*

4 ounces blackened chicken

1 cup cooked broccoli florets

1 whole-grain sandwich thin

2 tbsp light Italian dressing

DINNER

3½ ounces center-cut herb-seasoned
pork tenderloin

1 cup steamed green beans and ⅛ cup
slivered almonds

½ large baked potato (3–4¼ inches
in diameter)

1 tbsp olive oil

SNACK

1 medium orange

14 walnuts, halved

## Women's (135 Pounds) Meal Plan, Weeks 3–4

## Day 1

BREAKFAST

7 raw almonds

1 blueberry high-fiber waffle
with butter spray and calorie-free
syrup

*Blended Smoothie*

¼ cup frozen blueberries

1 scoop whey protein

ice and water

1 cup halved fresh strawberries

LUNCH

*Chef Salad*

¾ cup diced extra-lean ham

3 cups romaine lettuce

1 large, hard-boiled egg

balsamic vinegar and 2 tbsp light
ranch dressing


2 slices reduced-calorie wheat toast
with butter spray

1 medium apple, sliced

DINNER

4 ounces blackened salmon

½ cup couscous

10 small asparagus spears, steamed,
with 1 tbsp olive oil

**SNACK**

*Turkey Wrap*

1 multi-grain, high-fiber, low-calorie
  wrap

2 ounces roasted turkey breast
  (low sodium)

1 extra-small banana (less than 6 inches)

**POST-WORKOUT**

8 ounces Gatorade with 1 scoop
  whey protein

## Day 2

**BREAKFAST**

*Breakfast Wrap*

1 multi-grain, high-fiber, low-calorie
  wrap

½ cup egg whites and 1 whole egg

⅛ cup steamed spinach

hot sauce

1 cup fresh honeydew/cantaloupe

**LUNCH**

4 ounces basil and garlic shrimp

1 cup spaghetti squash

½ cup chopped red/green pepper

1 cup broccoli, chopped, cooked, with
  1 tbsp olive oil

**DINNER**

4 ounces Jamaican jerk chicken

½ cup brown rice

1 cup green beans, steamed

1 tbsp and 2 tsp olive oil

**SNACK**

5 raw almonds

*Blended Smoothie*

1 scoop whey protein

ice and water

½ cup pineapple chunks (in own juice)

1 cup raspberries

**POST-WORKOUT**

8 ounces Gatorade with 1 scoop
  whey protein

## Day 3

**BREAKFAST**

*Vanilla Peach Oatmeal*

½ cup oatmeal

½ cup sliced peaches

cinnamon and non-calorie sweetener

1 scoop vanilla whey protein

**LUNCH**

4 ounces beef tenderloin

1 small baked potato

1½ cups mixed roasted zucchini, squash,
  and red pepper, cooked with 2 tbsp
  olive oil

**DINNER**

4 ounces grouper, broiled, topped with
  ⅛ cup mango salsa

¼ cup brown rice

1½ cups steamed green/yellow
    bean mix

## SNACK

*Berry-Chocolate Yogurt*

6 ounces nonfat plain Greek yogurt

½ cup halved strawberries

1 tbsp ground flaxseed

1–2 tsp unsweetened cocoa

non-calorie sweetener

## POST-WORKOUT

8 ounces Gatorade with 1 scoop
    whey protein

## Day 4

### BREAKFAST

*Breakfast Sandwich*

1 egg and ½ cup egg substitute

⅛ cup shredded nonfat cheddar cheese

1 whole-grain English muffin

¼ cup chopped onion, cooked

¼ cup chopped pepper, cooked

2 tsp olive oil

### LUNCH

*Grilled Chicken Salad*

4 ounces grilled chicken, chopped

1 cup cherry tomatoes

¼ cup shredded carrots

½ cup chopped cucumber

3 cups romaine lettuce

2 tbsp light BBQ sauce

1 tbsp light ranch dressing

1 slice reduced-calorie wheat bread with
    butter spray

## DINNER

4 ounces grilled salmon with lemon

1 small sweet potato with butter spray,
    cinnamon, non-calorie sweetener

10 pecans, halved

1½ cups mixed vegetables (broccoli,
    cauliflower, carrots), cooked with
    2 tsp olive oil

## SNACK

13 raw almonds

*Blended Smoothie*

8 ounces nonfat skim milk

1 extra-small banana (less than 6 inches)

## POST-WORKOUT

8 ounces Gatorade with 1 scoop
    whey protein

## Day 5

### BREAKFAST

⅓ cup oatmeal with cinnamon and
    non-calorie sweetener

8 ounces nonfat plain Greek yogurt
    with 1 cup strawberries and non-
    calorie sweetener

10 raw almonds

LUNCH

*Sesame Chicken Salad*

3½ ounces chicken, sliced

3 cups fresh spinach

1 orange

½ cup alfalfa sprouts

2 tbsp sesame ginger dressing

1 tbsp sesame seeds, toasted

1 slice reduced-calorie wheat bread with
   butter spray

DINNER

*Shrimp Stir-fry*

4 ounces shrimp

½ cup brown rice

2 cups mixed Asian vegetables

rice vinegar

1½ tsp sesame seeds, toasted

ginger/desired spice

1 tbsp olive oil

SNACK

*Blended Smoothie*

½ scoop whey protein

8 ounces nonfat milk

ice

POST-WORKOUT

8 ounces Gatorade with 1 scoop whey
   protein

## Day 6

BREAKFAST

*Blended Smoothie*

¾ cup strawberries

1 scoop chocolate whey protein

1 whole-grain English muffin with 2
   tbsp peanut butter

LUNCH

*Steak Tacos*

3 ounces sirloin

2 small corn tortillas (4½ inches)

2 cups shredded romaine lettuce

¼ cup salsa

¼ cup shredded nonfat mozzarella
   cheese

¼ avocado

DINNER

*Chicken Stir-fry*

3½ ounces chicken

½ cup pineapple chunks

½ cup chopped bell pepper

½ cup brown rice

1 tbsp olive oil

SNACK

3 ounces nonfat plain Greek yogurt
   mixed with ranch powdered dip

20 baby carrots

## Day 7

**BREAKFAST**

½ cup oatmeal

*Egg Scramble*

½ cup egg substitute

¼ cup shredded nonfat cheddar
cheese

¾ cup cooked chopped spinach,
mushrooms, and tomato

1 tbsp olive oil

**LUNCH**

*Turkey Sandwich*

4 ounces oven roasted turkey

2 slices reduced-calorie wheat bread

1 lettuce leaf

1 tomato

yellow mustard

1 cup broccoli, steamed, with 1 tbsp
low-fat ranch dressing

**DINNER**

3½ ounces blackened chicken

3 ounces roasted red potatoes with
garlic

20 raw almonds

1 cup steamed green beans

**SNACK**

6 ounces nonfat plain Greek yogurt
mixed with non-calorie sweetener

1 cup halved fresh strawberries

1 ounce pistachio nuts

# Women's (135 Pounds) Meal Plan, Weeks 5–6

## Day 1

**BREAKFAST**

*Breakfast Sandwich*

3 ounces sliced Canadian bacon

1 hard-boiled egg

1 whole-wheat English muffin

5 sprays butter substitute

½ orange (3 inches in diameter)

**LUNCH**

*Chicken Salad*

4 ounces grilled chicken breast

1 tbsp buffalo sauce marinade

3 cups shredded romaine lettuce

½ ounce shredded part-skim mozzarella
cheese

1 slice reduced-calorie wheat bread with
5 sprays butter substitute

1 small apple

**DINNER**

5 ounces shrimp with Jamaican jerk
spices (as desired)

½ cup brown rice

1 cup steamed green/yellow bean blend

2 tbsp olive oil

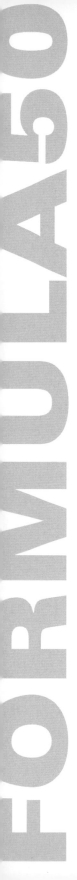

SNACK

8 ounces nonfat Greek yogurt
(any flavor)

5 raw almonds/walnuts

POST-WORKOUT

8 ounces Gatorade with 1 scoop
whey protein

## Day 2

BREAKFAST

7 raw almonds

1 whole-grain, high-fiber waffle with
butter spray and calorie-free syrup

*Blended Smoothie*

½ extra-small banana

1 scoop whey protein

ice and water

LUNCH

4 ounces grilled flank steak, with
garlic

1 medium sweet potato

1½ cups roasted zucchini and squash
with 1 tbsp olive oil

DINNER

4 ounces roast turkey with rosemary,
thyme, and basil

2 cups snap green beans and 10
almonds, sauteed in cooking
spray

2 pieces reduced-calorie bread with
2 tsp butter, whipped

SNACK

8 ounces nonfat milk with ½ scoop
whey protein

7 walnut halves

POST-WORKOUT

8 ounces Gatorade with 1 scoop whey
protein

## Day 3

BREAKFAST

*Breakfast Wrap*

1 multi-grain, high-fiber, low-calorie
wrap

1 cup egg whites/egg substitute

½ cup chopped fresh mushrooms

¼ cup steamed spinach

pepper-and-olive oil cooking spray

1 cup fresh honeydew/cantaloupe

LUNCH

3½ ounces pork tenderloin
with 2 tbsp chipotle pepper
marinade

*Dirty Rice*

½ cup brown rice

½ cup chopped jalapeno peppers

½ cup chopped onion

1 tbsp olive oil for flavor

nonfat cooking spray for saute

## DINNER

*Sesame Chicken*

4 ounces boneless, skinless chicken
    breast

1 tbsp Asian ginger marinade

1½ cups mixed Asian vegetables

½ cup couscous

1 tbsp sesame oil

1 tbsp sesame seeds

## SNACK

1 cup fresh raspberries

4 walnut halves

½ scoop whey protein mixed with water

## POST-WORKOUT

8 ounces Gatorade with 1 scoop whey
    protein

## Day 4

## BREAKFAST

1 whole-grain mini bagel with
    1 slice cheese

*Egg Scramble*

¼ cup chopped onion

½ cup chopped bell pepper

¾ cup egg whites

## LUNCH

*Hawaiian Chicken*

3½ ounces chicken tenderloin

3 tbsp low-calorie BBQ sauce

¼ cup pineapple chunks

¾ cup broccoli florets

½ cup wild rice

2 tsp olive oil

## DINNER

4 ounces blackened shrimp

½ medium potato with 1 tbsp whipped
    butter

1 cup cooked spinach with 1 tbsp
    olive oil

## SNACK

1 apple

24 raw almonds

6 ounces nonfat Greek yogurt
    (any flavor)

## POST-WORKOUT

8 ounces Gatorade with 1 scoop
    whey protein

## Day 5

## BREAKFAST

1 whole-grain, high-fiber waffle with
    1 tbsp creamy peanut butter

*Blended Smoothie*

1 scoop chocolate whey protein

½ small banana (6–7 inches)

ice and water

## LUNCH

*Tequila Lime Tilapia*

1 tbsp tequila lime seasoning

4 ounces grilled Tilapia

20 small asparagus spears (5 inches or less) with 1 tbsp olive oil

½ cup brown rice

## DINNER

*Beef Tacos*

4 ounces 96% lean ground beef

2 small corn tortillas (4½ inches)

2 cups shredded lettuce

¼ cup salsa

½ cup sliced plum tomatoes

½ cup chopped cucumber

## SNACK

8 ounces nonfat milk with 1 scoop whey protein

## POST-WORKOUT

8 ounces Gatorade with 1 scoop whey protein

## Day 6

## BREAKFAST

2 slices reduced-calorie bread with 2 tsp whole-fruit spread

4 (1-ounce) slices of Canadian bacon

2 eggs, sunny-side up

½ cup honeydew melon

## LUNCH

*Cheeseburger*

3½ ounces grilled 96% lean ground beef

1 slice nonfat cheese stuffed inside burger

¼-inch slice tomato

2 slices reduced-calorie wheat bread

*Salad*

3 cups romaine lettuce

2 tbsp fat-free Caesar dressing

## DINNER

4 ounces herb-crusted salmon topped with diced tomato and garlic

*Rice Pilaf*

½ cup brown rice

1 clove garlic

¼ cup finely chopped onion

1 tsp olive oil

## SNACK

*Blended Smoothie*

8 ounces nonfat milk

½ scoop vanilla whey protein

¼ cup mango

¼ extra-small banana (less than 6 inches)

## Day 7

### BREAKFAST

1 whole-wheat English muffin with
   1 tbsp peanut butter

*Blended Smoothie*

½ cup strawberries

1 scoop whey protein powder

ice and water

### LUNCH

4 ounces blackened mahi mahi
   (or other fish)

1 small baked potato with 10 sprays
   low-calorie butter spray and ½ ounce
   shredded cheese, part skim

1 cup mixed vegetables, roasted with
   garlic, cooked in 1 tbsp olive oil

### DINNER

*Mediterranean-Style Chicken*

4 ounces grilled chicken

1 cup diced, canned tomatoes

1 clove garlic

2 tbsp dried basil

1–2 tbsp diced olives

1 ounce grated Parmesan
   cheese

½ cup yellow rice, cooked, with ½ cup
   chopped green pepper with 2 tsp
   olive oil

### SNACK

8 ounces nonfat milk

½ cup strawberries

# 9

# Formula 50, the Advanced Plan

**Y**OU NEED A PLAN TO ACCOMPLISH GREAT FEATS, whether of physical strength or sheer will. I don't enter a studio without having written any songs and expect to have a No. 1 single to show for my poor preparation. I don't show up on the first day of a movie shoot clueless about the script, thinking I can just fake it when the director yells "action." Likewise, I don't wander into the gym and expect to transform my body by randomly picking up some weights and putting them down.

Fail to prepare and you prepare to fail, they say, and it's true. You need a fitness plan to become fit. Welcome to the advanced phase of Formula 50—training on a different level. I enter this mode when it's time to dial it in for an important movie, tour, or other event. My body rocks when I train this way. The results never cease to amaze me.

Here's the fitness equivalent of a warning label on a rap CD: *This isn't something the uninitiated can dive into without having first completed the beginner's phase.* If you're new to the gym, start with the beginner's program. I implore you. Complete those 6 weeks of training exactly as I break them down. Only then will you be ready for the advanced phase. Otherwise, you'll feel like a riot's broken out inside your body, and the chaotic demands will overwhelm your energy, hormonal, and musculoskeletal systems, all of which will start setting off alarms.

If you're already more experienced, you have the option of diving headfirst into the advanced phase. I suggest you go through the beginner's phase first, though, regardless of your experience level. If you haven't trained in this style before, it could take some adjustment. Because the beginner's workouts are so balanced and functional, they're also good for correcting any existing bad training habits. If you've been focusing on, say, curls or the bench press before, other parts of your body—especially smaller supporting muscles—may be neglected. The beginner's program will remedy that over 6 weeks, which will set you up for the additional 6 weeks of advanced work.

The workouts themselves are structured a little differently in this phase. The biggest changes between the beginner's phase and this one are (1) an additional day of energy system training; (2) more variety among resistance training sessions, especially during the final 3 weeks; and (3) shorter rest periods in between sets. You're rolling in these workouts. They'll push anyone to new heights of conditioning, both cardiovascular and muscular endurance.

Some of the exercises in the beginner's program are also used in the advanced program. It's not like there are "beginner" moves and "advanced" moves. Usually the changes relate more to intensity (weight lifted), volume (sets multiplied by reps), and rest periods (less rest is always more challenging). A lunge, for example, can tax a beginner, but it can be made to tax an advanced lifter. Despite the overlap, the advanced program includes some added spice in exercise selection, which makes it fun. If you're like me, you'll welcome a good challenge.

Six days of training for 6 weeks is very manageable. Doing this for 6 months instead of 6 weeks might result in overtraining. But with proper nutrition and plenty of rest, you can kill this program for the next month and a half, and look like a million bucks when you reach the end.

As you proceed through the advanced plan, you'll notice that the time spent working out will shrink in some cases. This simply reflects shorter rest periods. The workouts become shorter but harder. This is the most efficient training style there is, which is why I've embraced it. But your body will adjust to it in amazing ways, as will your mind. Your willpower is stronger than any muscle in your body, but it needs to be trained and developed as well.

In Week 7, when you're given only 30 seconds of rest between superset pairings, it'll seem short and rushed compared to when you had a minute's rest. But by the time your rest is down to 20 seconds, 30 seconds will seem like a breeze. Even when you're down to 10 seconds in between, time will slow as you maintain your focus. Those three deep breaths you have time to draw will seem like they last 3 minutes. Mind over matter. Will over won't. You'll hit the next set with more focus.

So are you ready? This is it. Make it through these next 6 weeks and you will have built the health-and-fitness foundation for the rest of your life.

## Phase 3: Weeks 7–9

| Week | Monday | Tuesday | Wednesday | Thursday | Friday | Saturday | Sunday |
|------|--------|---------|-----------|----------|--------|----------|--------|
| #7 | Strength 3-A | EST 3 | Strength 3-B | EST 3 | Strength 3-A | EST 3 | Off |
| #8 | Strength 3-B | EST 3 | Strength 3-A | EST 3 | Strength 3-B | EST 3 | Off |
| #9 | Strength 3-A | EST 3 | Strength 3-B | EST 3 | Strength 3-A | EST 3 | Off |

EST = Energy System Training

### EST 3

During these 3 weeks, each session should begin and end with a leisurely paced 3 to 5 minutes on a treadmill or other cardio apparatus. This is your warm-up and cool-down.

**Week 7:** You're going to do 6 intervals, going very hard for 1 minute before backing off to a slower pace for 2 minutes.

**Week 8:** Same drill, only I want you to squeeze out 7 intervals for me.

**Week 9:** Repeat, only I want you to squeeze out 8 intervals for me.

# STRENGTH 3-A

## Dynamic Warm-Up/Flexibility

| Exercise | Sets | Reps | Load | Tempo | Rest | Intensity |
|---|---|---|---|---|---|---|
| Spine Twist | 1 | 5/side | Body-weight | Moderate | None | Low |
| Kneeling Hip Opener | 1 | 5 | Body-weight | Moderate | None | Low |
| Twisting Lunge Stretch | 1 | 5/side | Body-weight | Moderate | None | Low |
| Side Squat | 1 | 5/side | Body-weight | Moderate | None | Low |

## Activation Drills

| Drill | Sets | Reps | Load | Tempo[1] | Rest | Intensity |
|---|---|---|---|---|---|---|
| Lateral Walk | 1 | 10–12/side | Body-weight | 2011 | None | Low |
| Wall Slide | 1 | 10 | Body-weight | 2011 | None | Low |

## Strength Training

| Exercise | Sets[2] | Reps | Load[3] | Tempo[1] | Rest (secs) | Intensity |
|---|---|---|---|---|---|---|
| A1. Split Squat | 3 | 8–10/side | TBD | 3010 | 30, 20, 10 | High |
| A2. Bench Press | 3 | 8–10 | TBD | 3010 | 30, 20, 10 | High |
| A3. Stationary Bike | 3 | 60 seconds | N/A | Fast | 60, 60, 60 | High |
| B1. Romanian Dead Lift | 3 | 8–10 | TBD | 3010 | 30, 20, 10 | High |
| B2. Seated Row | 3 | 8–10 | TBD | 3010 | 30, 20, 10 | High |
| B3. Stationary Bike | 3 | 60 seconds | N/A | Fast | 60, 60, 60 | High |
| C1. Dip | 3 | 8–10 | Body-weight | 3010 | 30, 20, 10 | High |
| C2. Ball Rollout | 3 | 8–10 | Body-weight | 2020 | 30, 20, 10 | High |
| C3. Stationary Bike | 3 | 60 seconds | N/A | Fast | 60, 60, 60 | High |

[1] "Tempo" refers to the speed of movement. For example, 3-1-1-0 means: 3 seconds lowering the weight; 1 second pause in the lengthened position; 1 second to raise the weight; no pause ("0") in the contracted position.

[2] When you see exercises preceded by the same letter, complete those sets before moving on to the next pairing. For example, in Week 7, do 1 set of split squats (A1), rest 30 seconds, do a set of bench presses (A2), rest 30 seconds, spend 60 seconds on the bike (A3), and then rest 60 seconds. Only after finishing all 3 sets of all 3 exercises do you proceed to the next pairing (B, in this case). Perform those sets in the same consecutive fashion.

[3] Choose a weight at which you fail in the desired rep range. For the bench press, if you can do only 7 reps, your weight is too heavy. If you can do 11, it's too light. Adjust your weight selection accordingly.

**Flexibility training:** Perform immediately post-workout. See Chapter 6, page 61, for details.

**Foam rolling:** Perform immediately after stretching. See Chapter 6, page 72, for details.

## DYNAMIC WARM-UP/FLEXIBILITY

1. **Spine Twist**

   See Chapter 7, page 103, for description.

2. **Kneeling Hip Opener**

   See Chapter 7, page 104, for description.

3. **Twisting Lunge Stretch**

   See Chapter 7, page 105, for description.

4. **Side Squat**

   See Chapter 7, page 106, for description.

## ACTIVATION DRILLS

1. **Lateral Walk**

   See Chapter 7, page 107, for description.

2. **Wall Slide,** see below.

**BASIC MOVE**
# Wall Slide

**PURPOSE** | This stretch helps you open your shoulders, encouraging you to retract your scapulae, which is necessary for getting the most out of exercises that work your chest, shoulder, and back muscles.

**GET READY** | Stand with your back flat against a wall. Place your hands above your head so that your elbows, wrists, and the back of your hands are against the wall. Your upper arms should form 90-degree angles with your torso, and your forearms should make 90-degree angles with your upper arms.

**GO** | While holding your shoulders down, slide your arms up along the wall, keeping the backs of your hands, wrists, and elbows in contact with the wall. If any of these parts of your body begin to lose contact, stop raising your arms. Reverse the action

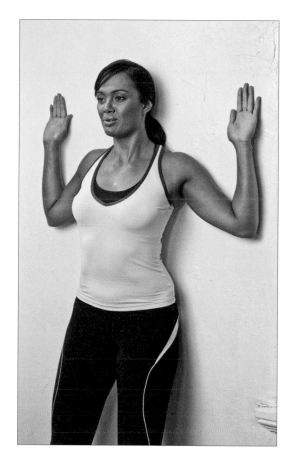
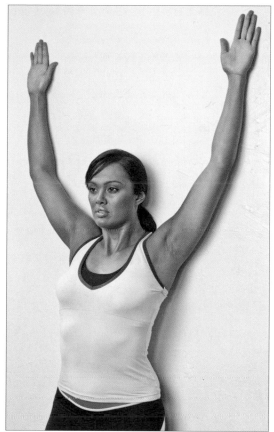

by bringing your arms down and your elbows below your shoulders and in toward your body as much as you can while maintaining those same points of contact the entire time. Make sure that you keep your shoulder blades together and against the wall throughout the set. You may feel tightness in your mid-back and a stretch in the front of your shoulders. Perform this move at a slow, deliberate pace for the given number of reps.

**FIFTY SAYS** | "If your shoulders are tight, then this is harder than it looks. It's a crucial move for opening up your shoulders and other upper-body muscles for better growth without injury."

STRENGTH TRAINING

## BASIC MOVE
## Split Squat

See Chapter 7, page 94, for description.

## BASIC MOVE
## Bench Press

**SPECIAL FEATURES** | Barbell, incline bench

**TARGET** | Pectorals, triceps, front delts

**PURPOSE** | While the bench press is a compound movement that primarily targets the pectorals, this exercise also requires help from the triceps and shoulders.

**GET READY** | Lie on an incline bench with your feet planted firmly on the ground. Using a medium-width grip (slightly wider than your shoulders), hold it straight over your upper chest with your arms fully extended. Keep your shoulders down and back at the start and throughout the set.

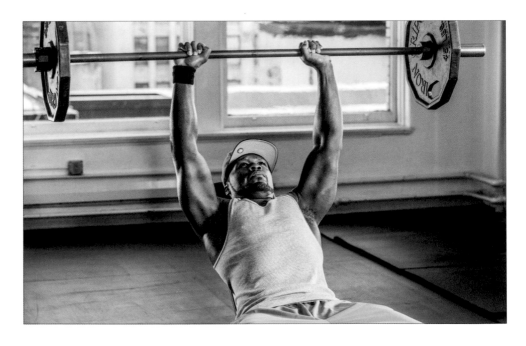

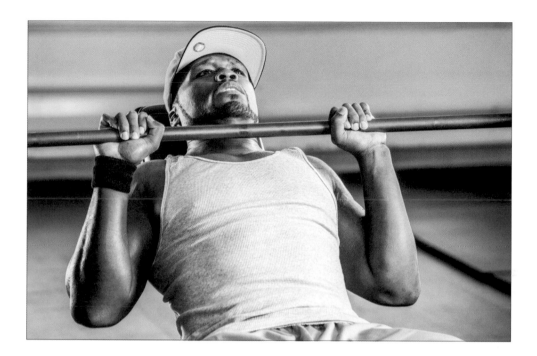

**GO** | Lower the bar with control, stretching your pecs. Take the bar down until it touches your chest, and feel the stretch, keeping your pectorals engaged through the entire range of motion. Each upper arm should form a 45-degree angle with your torso at this point in the movement. Press the bar up until your arms are fully extended, emphasizing the contraction in your arm muscles.

**FIFTY SAYS** | "To get the most from barbell bench presses, avoid shifting your body or moving your shoulders while you're performing the set. Keep the action in your chest at all times. Lock in, and stretch and contract your pecs to move the weight. Again: quality over quantity."

# Stationary Bike

**SPECIAL FEATURES** | Fan bike (if available)

**TARGET** | Legs, cardiovascular, fat burning

**PURPOSE** | To increase your heart rate and tap into body fat, burning it as energy.

**GET READY** | Adjust the seat of a fan or stationary bike so that your legs approach full extension at the bottom of each revolution. At no time should your knees "lock out" during the set. Place the balls of your feet on the pedals and grasp the handles. Keep your torso upright throughout the set.

**GO** | Pedal hard for the length of time listed in the chart, pumping your arms and legs (if a fan bike is available). Your perceived rate of exertion should reach about 9 out of 10 for most of the set. Push it.

**FIFTY SAYS** | "Fan bikes take the intensity to a whole new level compared to other stationary bikes, so use one if it's available. If not, then opt for an upright stationary bike over a recumbent one."

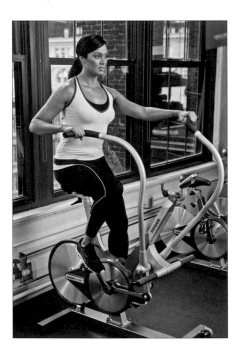
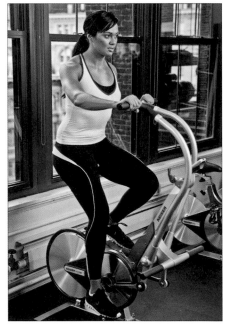

# Romanian Dead Lift

**SPECIAL FEATURES** | Dumbbells

**TARGET** | Hamstrings, glutes, lower back

**PURPOSE** | Romanian dead lifts provide intense muscular stimulation for your hips and glutes while removing your quads from the action.

**GET READY** | Stand tall with your feet about hip-width apart, your chest up, and your shoulders down. With your knees slightly bent, place a pair of dumbbells on or in front of your thighs with your palms facing your body.

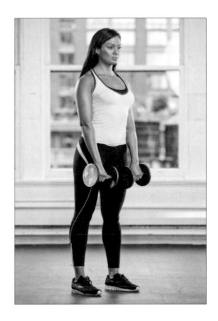

**GO** | Holding the natural curve in your lower back throughout the set, begin to bend at the hips, pressing them back as you continue to hold the same bend at your knees while performing all reps. As you lower the dumbbells, keep them close to the front of your legs. You should feel a stretch in your hamstrings and glutes as you reach the bottom of the movement. Reverse the motion, pulling your hips forward as you stand upright. Keep your back in its neutral position, your chest forward, and your shoulders down and back as you perform the set.

**FIFTY SAYS** | "Don't just bend over when you're doing this move. It's important that you push your hips back to deepen the work of your target muscles."

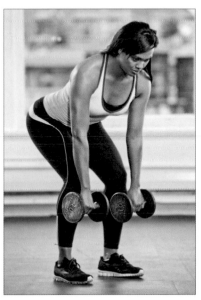

# Seated Row

**SPECIAL FEATURES** | Cable, split-handle, pronated grip, elbows out

**TARGET** | Lats, upper-back muscles

**PURPOSE** | To encourage the development of the small muscles of the upper back.

**GET READY** | Choose your weight and sit on the bench of a seated row setup. Grasp the handle with both hands and, with your arms straight, pull the weights an inch or two off the stack. Your feet should be planted firmly on the platform with a slight bend in your knees. Keep your torso tall, chest lifted, and shoulders down. Elevate your upper arms and wrists so that your arms are parallel to the floor. Tighten your core before you begin the action of the set.

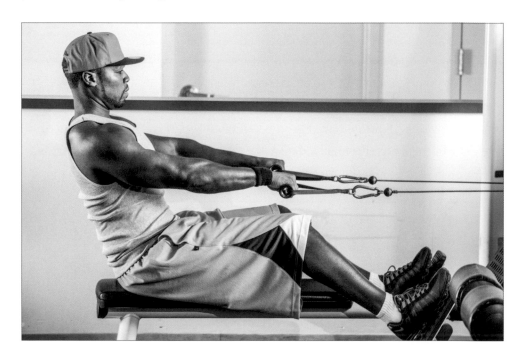

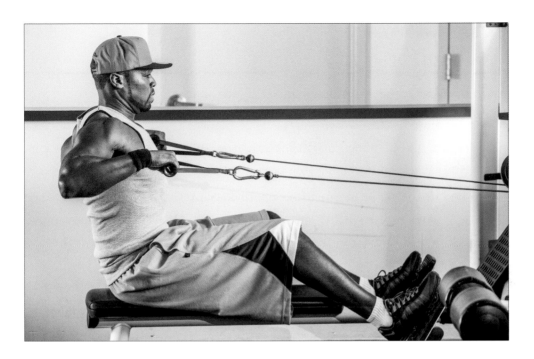

**GO** | Pull the weight toward your chest until your elbows are just behind your shoulders. Keep your torso stationary throughout the set. You should feel the stretch and flex in the muscles of your upper back.

**FIFTY SAYS** | "You don't want to let your upper body bend forward or back when you're moving the weights on this move, because that undercuts the amount of detail you're able to sear into the muscles of your upper back. Also, remember that the higher you pull the weight into your body, the more you emphasize the muscles of your upper back."

# Stationary Bike

See page 156 for description.

**BASIC MOVE**

# Dip

**SPECIAL FEATURES** | Standard

**TARGET** | Triceps, pecs

**PURPOSE** | To build muscular, detailed triceps. This move also recruits key supporting muscle groups, including your pecs and shoulders.

**GET READY** | Start at the top of the dip. To do this, take a hold of the dip bars and jump or press yourself up so that your arms are straight, perpendicular to the ground. Hold your shoulders down and chest up. Bend your legs and cross your ankles behind you. Make sure your wrist joints aren't bent.

**GO** | Bend your arms to lower your torso. Your elbows should travel behind your back rather than flaring out to your sides. Feel a stretch along the top of your upper

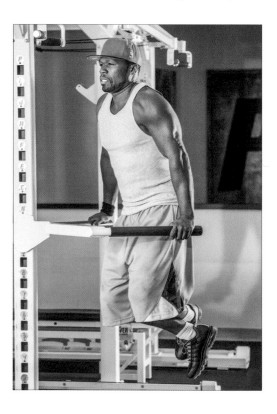
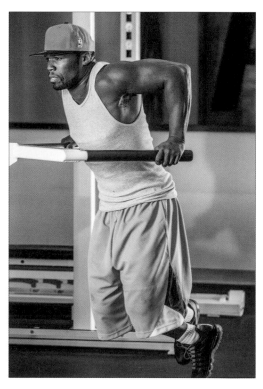

arms in your triceps. Go as low as you can without feeling any pain in your shoulder joints; typically, your upper arms should be parallel to the ground at the bottom of the movement. Keeping your chest up, shoulders back and eyes looking forward, press your body up, contracting your triceps and chest. At the top of the move, force a contraction into your triceps, but avoid locking out your elbows. Keep the move deliberate and steady throughout the set.

**FIFTY SAYS** | "You see a lot of guys bouncing up and down as fast as they can when they're performing dips, trying to get as many reps as they can. But that wrecks your shoulders and undercuts the work you want your triceps to perform. This move is also about quality, not quantity."

**BASIC MOVE**
# Ball Rollout

See Chapter 7, page 114, for description.

**BASIC MOVE**
# Stationary Bike

See page 156 for description.

## STRENGTH 3-B

### Dynamic Warm-Up/Flexibility

| Exercise | Sets | Reps | Load | Tempo | Rest | Intensity |
|---|---|---|---|---|---|---|
| Spine Twist | 1 | 5/side | Body-weight | Moderate | None | Low |
| Kneeling Hip Opener | 1 | 5 | Body-weight | Moderate | None | Low |
| Twisting Lunge Stretch | 1 | 5/side | Body-weight | Moderate | None | Low |
| Side Squat | 1 | 5/side | Body-weight | Moderate | None | Low |

### Activation Drills

| Drill | Sets | Reps | Load | Tempo[1] | Rest | Intensity |
|---|---|---|---|---|---|---|
| Lateral Walk | 1 | 10–12/side | Body-weight | 2011 | None | Low |
| Wall Slide | 1 | 10 | Body-weight | 2011 | None | Low |

### Exercises

| Exercise | Sets[2] | Reps | Load[3] | Tempo[1] | Rest (secs) | Intensity |
|---|---|---|---|---|---|---|
| A1. Dead Lift | 3 | 8–10 | TBD | 3010 | 30, 20, 10 | High |
| A2. Bench Press | 3 | 8–10 | TBD | 3010 | 30, 20, 10 | High |
| A3. VersaClimber | 3 | 60 seconds | N/A | Fast | 60, 60, 60 | High |
| B1. Side Lunge | 3 | 8–10/side | TBD | 3010 | 30, 20, 10 | High |
| B2. Chin-Up | 3 | 8–10 | TBD | 3010 | 30, 20, 10 | High |
| B3. Rowing Machine | 3 | 60 seconds | N/A | Fast | 60, 60, 60 | High |
| C1. Biceps Curl | 3 | 8–10 | Body-weight | 3010 | 30, 20, 10 | High |
| C2. Suitcase Walk | 3 | 10–12/side | Body-weight | Moderate | 30, 20, 10 | High |
| C3. Stationary Bike | 3 | 60 seconds | N/A | Fast | 60, 60, 60 | High |

[1] "Tempo" refers to the speed of movement. For example, 3-1-1-0 means: 3 seconds lowering the weight; 1 second pause in the lengthened position; 1 second to raise the weight; no pause ("0") in the contracted position.

[2] When you see exercises preceded by the same letter, complete those sets before moving on to the next pairing. For example, in Week 7, do 1 set of dead lifts (A1), rest 30 seconds, do a set of incline bench presses (A2), rest 30 seconds, spend 60 seconds on the VersaClimber (A3), and then rest 60 seconds. Only after finishing all 3 sets of all 3 exercises do you proceed to the next pairing (B, in this case). Perform those sets in the same consecutive fashion.

[3] Choose a weight at which you fail in the desired rep range. For the incline bench press, if you can do only 7 reps, your weight is too heavy. If you can do 11, it's too light. Adjust your weight selection accordingly.

**Flexibility training:** Perform immediately post-workout. See Chapter 6, page 61, for details.

**Foam rolling:** Perform immediately after stretching. See Chapter 6, page 72, for details.

## DYNAMIC WARM-UP/FLEXIBILITY

1. **Spine Twist**

   See Chapter 7, page 103, for description.

2. **Kneeling Hip Opener**

   See Chapter 7, page 104, for description.

3. **Twisting Lunge Stretch**

   See Chapter 7, page 105, for description.

4. **Side Squat**

   See Chapter 7, page 106, for description.

## ACTIVATION DRILLS

1. **Lateral Walk**

   See Chapter 7, page 107, for description.

2. **Wall Slide**

   See page 152 for description.

## STRENGTH TRAINING

**BASIC MOVE**

# Dead Lift

**SPECIAL FEATURES** | Barbell, clean grip

**TARGET** | Legs, lower back

**PURPOSE** | To stimulate overall muscle growth with an emphasis on the lower body and lower back.

**GET READY** | Load a bar with the desired amount of weight and place it on the ground. Step up to it, placing your toes under the bar (elevated off the ground by the weight plates) with your shins close to the bar. Your feet should be hip-width apart. Bend at the hips and knees and grip the bar with an overhand grip (palms facing you). Your hands should be shoulder-width apart. Before beginning the set, shift your weight onto your heels, lift your chest up, and pull your shoulders back and down.

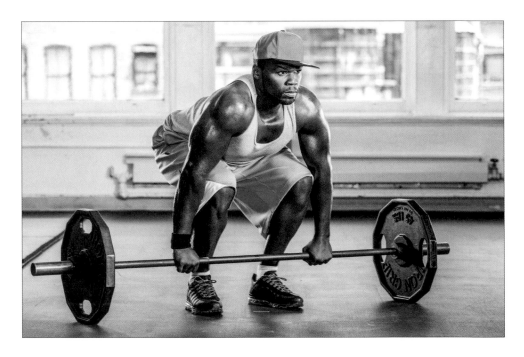

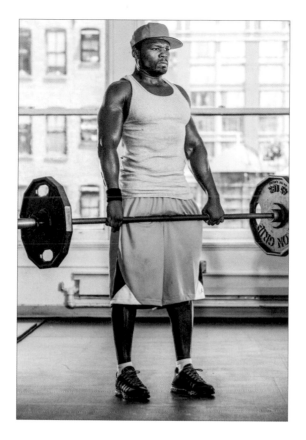

**GO** | Pull the weight straight up, beginning by driving through your heels. Continue to move the weight by contracting your glutes and core muscles, straightening your legs at the knee joint. Finish the lift by pressing your hips forward until you're standing fully upright. Reverse the motion by bending only at the hips, keeping the barbell close to your hips. Begin to bend your knees as the weight lowers to them. Place the weight back on the ground. Pause at the bottom for a second, checking your body position before you begin the next rep. Your back should be flat throughout the set.

**FIFTY SAYS** | "I like the rhythm and effort this move requires. I think of each rep as being performed in two phases. First you straighten your lower legs at the knees, then you straighten your body at the hips. When you lower the weight, you use the reverse rhythm."

# Bench Press

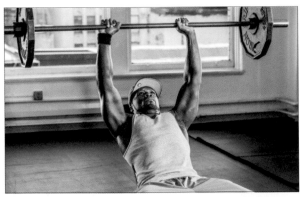

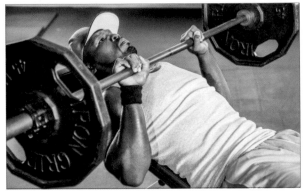

**SPECIAL FEATURES** | Incline, barbell

**TARGET** | Chest

**PURPOSE** | This variation on the standard barbell bench press recruits more muscle fibers in the upper pectorals, helping you achieve a fuller chest.

**GET READY** | Set a bench at about a 30-degree incline (the standard angle of many fixed inclined barbell benches) and place the desired amount of weight on the barbell. Lie on the bench and take hold of the barbell with an overhand grip, placing your hands a little wider than your shoulders. Unrack the bar by extending your arms and hold it above your sternum, pulling your shoulders back and down.

**GO** | Lower the bar so that your upper arms flare out, forming 45-degree angles with your torso. Think about pulling the weight down to your upper chest, maintaining strict control throughout. Feel that stretch across your upper chest. Then, without transferring the effort out of your pecs, press the weight up through the same range of motion. Hold your shoulders back and contract your pecs at the top of the movement. Also, avoid locking your elbows at the top of the movement.

**FIFTY SAYS** | "Avoid resting between or during reps by shifting the weight into your shoulders. Keep your pecs active throughout the whole set to get the most from this exercise."

# VersaClimber

**SPECIAL FEATURES** | Standard

**TARGET** | Legs, upper body, cardiovascular, fat burning

**PURPOSE** | To engage your whole body, elevating your heart rate and encouraging a higher metabolic rate for more fat burning.

**GET READY** | Place each of your feet on a pedal of the VersaClimber and adjust the straps so that your feet are comfortably secured. You should not be able to lift your feet off the pedals. Grab the handles on either side of the VersaClimber. Hold your torso upright, maintaining the natural curve in your lower back throughout the set.

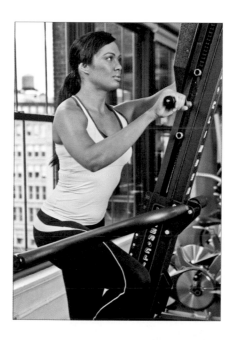

**GO** | Start the movement by simultaneously driving your same-side knee and arm up the track as you lower your other-side knee and arm, sliding the handles and pedals up and down the track. Make sure you hold your core tight and refrain from jerking your body up and down; keep the movement smooth throughout. Take small quick pumps with your limbs, and make sure your chest is up and your eyes are looking straight ahead. Continue the movement, making it as intense as you can, for the given time period.

**FIFTY SAYS** | "Performing your intense cardio sessions on various types of equipment helps create muscle confusion to make your body work even harder, burning body fat more effectively. Like a good DJ, a good workout should mix it up!"

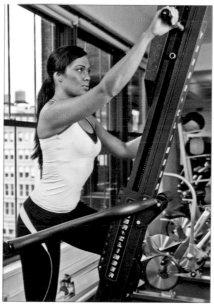

## BASIC MOVE
# Side Lunge

**SPECIAL FEATURES** | Body weight

**TARGET** | Glutes, quads, adductors, hamstrings

**PURPOSE** | This move works many muscles in your legs, but it especially targets the smaller muscles on the inside of your upper legs; it's a great move for encouraging overall leg development and improving conditioning and performance in many sports. It's also great for supplementing squats, lunges, and other lower-body moves that directly target larger leg muscles.

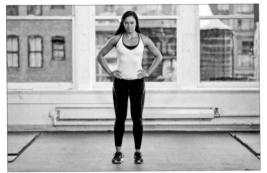

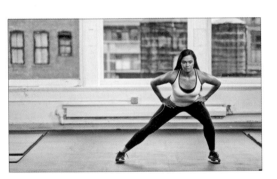

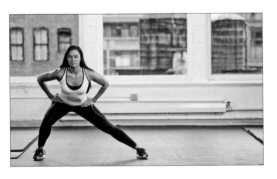

**GET READY** | Stand tall with your feet shoulder-width apart.

**GO** | Step 2 to 3 feet to the side with one foot. Bend at that knee and lower your hips toward the foot that you just moved, keeping your other leg straight. As you lower, load your body weight onto the heel of your bent leg, keeping your hips down and back. Make sure that both feet stay on the ground with your toes facing forward. Push through your bent leg to return to the starting position. Alternate legs, repeating until you've completed all reps.

**FIFTY SAYS** | "After your body is accustomed to the range of motion using body weight, you can progress to holding dumbbells as you perform the set, increasing the work your target muscles must perform."

# Chin-Up

**SPECIAL FEATURES** | Neutral grip, shoulder-width hand placement

**TARGET** | Lats

**PURPOSE** | Chin-ups are a great companion move to overhand-grip pull-ups. Chin-ups give your lats a deeper stretch and contraction as you move through a range of motion greater than what standard pull-ups allow.

**GET READY** | Take hold of the parallel bars on a set of pull-up bars. Use a neutral grip with your palms facing each other. Let your body hang with your arms straight.

**GO** | Start the movement by drawing your shoulder blades together and opening your chest. Lean back and pull your chest up, keeping your shoulders down and your neck relaxed throughout the set. Feel a contraction in your back at the top of the movement. Slowly lower yourself back to the starting position. Keep the focus on your back as you descend, feeling a stretch. Keep the movement smooth throughout; try not to jerk your body or buck your hips to assist you.

**FIFTY SAYS** | "If your gym doesn't have parallel bars attached to the pull-up bar, perform your chin-ups using the pull-up portion of the bar, with your palms rotated so that they face your body."

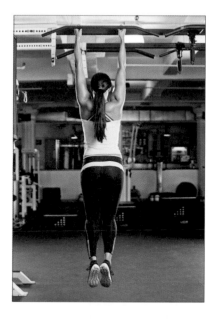

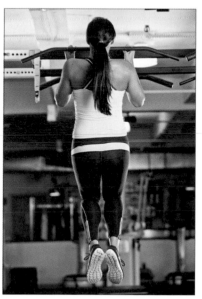

## BASIC MOVE
# Rowing Machine

**SPECIAL FEATURES** | Mechanical fan

**TARGET** | Legs, back, cardiovascular, fat burning

**PURPOSE** | To incorporate both lower- and upper-body work into intense cardiovascular work to promote efficient fat burning.

**GET READY** | Sit on the machine's sliding seat pad and secure your feet in the stirrups. Bend your knees, grab the handle with both hands, and release it from its catch. Make sure that your shoulders are down and your back is flat.

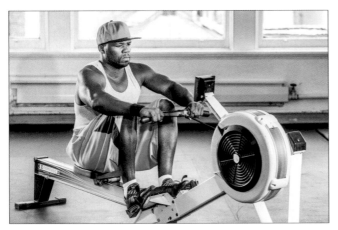

**GO** | Without moving your back or arms, begin by driving your legs. As your legs extend, lean back a bit (still maintaining the natural curve of your spine), and pull the handle to your lower chest. Keep your shoulders down and chest up. Straighten your arms and bend your legs to slide the seat close to the mechanical fan.

**FIFTY SAYS** | "Once I know how many meters I row for my baseline time, I'll sometimes row for that distance, trying to do it as fast as I can to beat my record time."

# Biceps Curl

See Chapter 7, page 120, for description.

# Suitcase Walk

**SPECIAL FEATURES** | Dumbbell

**TARGET** | Grip, shoulders, stabilizers

**PURPOSE** | This move works your body in an unbalanced way with a heavy load. You can thank me the next time you need to hustle a suitcase through an airport to catch a connecting flight. It's also beneficial training for those sports where stuff is coming at you from all different directions—in other words, most sports.

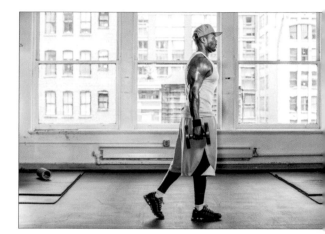

**GET READY** | Help yourself to a heavy dumbbell. Hold it at the side of your body with your palm facing your body and your arm hanging straight. Your chest should be up and open. Your shoulders will sag a bit, but try to keep them at the same height throughout the set, despite the hunk of metal dangling on one side.

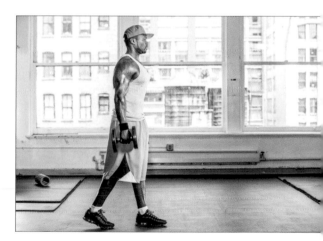

**GO** | Brace your core. Grasp that dumbbell as if you want to choke that sucker. Begin striding forward, making sure your torso doesn't sway to either side. Complete the prescribed number of steps/reps with the dumbbell in one hand before passing it to the other hand. Maintain proper posture and a firm grip on the dumbbell throughout the set.

**FIFTY SAYS** | "This is a great exercise that helps you perform better in many sports and at the gym, and it helps prep you for long hauls through airports if you travel frequently with heavy carry-on bags."

BASIC MOVE
# Stationary Bike

See page 158 for description.

## Phase 4: Weeks 10–12

| Week | Monday | Tuesday | Wednesday | Thursday | Friday | Saturday | Sunday |
|------|--------|---------|-----------|----------|--------|----------|--------|
| #10 | Strength 4-A | EST 4 | Strength 4-B | EST 4 | Strength 4-C | EST 4 | Off |
| #11 | Strength 4-A | EST 4 | Strength 4-B | EST 4 | Strength 4-C | EST 4 | Off |
| #12 | Strength 4-A | EST 4 | Strength 4-B | EST 4 | Strength 4-C | EST 4 | Off |

EST = Energy System Training

### EST 4

During these 3 weeks, each session should begin and end with a leisurely paced 3 to 5 minutes on a treadmill or other cardio apparatus. This is your warm-up and cool-down.

**Week 10:** You're going to do 8 intervals, going way hard for 30 seconds before backing off to a slower pace for 90 seconds.

**Week 11:** Same drill, only squeeze out 9 intervals for me.

**Week 12:** Same drill, only squeeze out 10 intervals for me.

# STRENGTH 4-A

## Dynamic Warm-Up/Flexibility

| Exercise | Sets | Reps | Load | Tempo | Rest | Intensity |
|---|---|---|---|---|---|---|
| Side-Lying Spinal Twist | 1 | 5/side | Body-weight | Moderate | None | Low |
| Hip Flexor Stretch | 1 | 5/side | Body-weight | Moderate | None | Low |
| Twisting Lunge Stretch | 1 | 5/side | Body-weight | Moderate | None | Low |
| Drop Step Lunge | 1 | 5/side | Body-weight | Moderate | None | Low |

## Activation Drills

| Drill | Sets | Reps | Load | Tempo[1] | Rest | Intensity |
|---|---|---|---|---|---|---|
| Lateral Walk | 1 | 10–12/side | Body-weight | 2011 | None | Low |
| Wall Slide | 1 | 10 | Body-weight | 2011 | None | Low |

## Strength Training

| Exercise | Sets[2] | Reps | Load[3] | Tempo[1] | Rest (secs) | Intensity |
|---|---|---|---|---|---|---|
| A1. Dead Lift | 3–4 | 8–10 | TBD | 3010 | 30, 20, 10 | High |
| A2. Bench Press | 3–4 | 8–10 | TBD | 3010 | 30, 20, 10 | High |
| A3. Hip Bridge | 3–4 | 8–10/side | TBD | 3010 | 30, 20, 10 | High |
| A4. Chin-Up | 3–4 | 8–10 | Body-weight | 3010 | 30, 20, 10 | High |
| A5. Prowler Push | 3–4 | 150 feet | TBD | 3010 | 30, 20, 10 | High |
| A6. Hammer Curl | 3–4 | 8–10 | TBD | 3010 | 30, 20, 10 | High |
| A7. Triceps Extension | 3–4 | 8–10 | TBD | 3010 | 30, 20, 10 | High |
| A8. Reverse Crunch | 3–4 | 8–10 | Body-weight | 2020 | 120 | High |

[1] "Tempo" refers to the speed of movement. For example, 3-1-1-0 means: 3 seconds lowering the weight; 1 second pause in the lengthened position; 1 second to raise the weight; no pause ("0") in the contracted position.

[2] Perform each exercise, all 8 of 'em, in succession, resting 30 seconds between each one, at least during Week 10. At the end of A8 (the reverse crunch), rest 120 seconds. You'll need it. Then repeat the circuit again under the same scenario, until you've completed 3 circuits—4 only if you can handle it.

During Week 11, decrease your rest in between moves to 20 seconds while keeping the 120-second break at the end of each circuit. During Week 12, decrease it to 10 seconds—barely time to suck down a few gulps of air.

[3] Choose a weight at which you fail in the desired rep range. On the bench press, for example, if you can bang out only 7 reps, lighten your load. If you can do 11, though, it's too light. Adjust your weight selection accordingly.

**Flexibility training:** Perform immediately post-workout. See Chapter 6, page 61, for details.

**Foam rolling:** Perform immediately after stretching. See Chapter 6, page 72, for details.

### DYNAMIC WARM-UP/FLEXIBILITY

1. **Side-Lying Spinal Twist**

   See Chapter 7, page 88, for description.

2. **Hip Flexor Stretch**

   See Chapter 7, page 90, for description.

3. **Twisting Lunge Stretch**

   See Chapter 7, page 105, for description.

4. **Drop Step Lunge**, see below.

**BASIC MOVE**

# Drop Step Lunge

**PURPOSE** | To open your hip and knee joints, and warm up your body.

**GET READY** | Stand tall with your feet hip-width apart and your chest up.

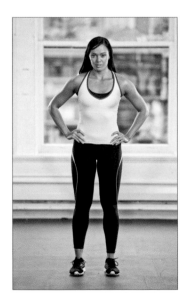

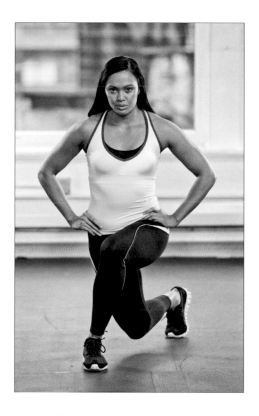 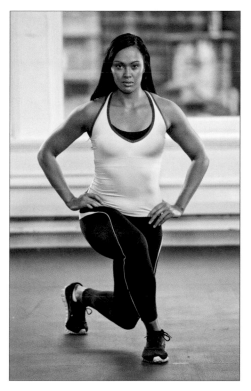

**GO** | Step your right foot back and about 2 feet to the left of your left foot. Once your back foot contacts the ground, square your hips, chest, and feet so they all face forward. Bend at the knees and sit back slowly, dropping your back knee toward the ground. Feel the stretch in the outside of your thigh and glutes. Keep your chest up and body squared, facing forward the entire time. Stand up, pressing through your back foot to return to the starting position. Repeat on the other side. Continue alternating until you've completed all reps.

**FIFTY SAYS** | "This is a great move for opening your knee and hip joints from your backside, and it's another move you can perform anytime, anyplace."

## ACTIVATION DRILLS

1. **Lateral Walk**

   See Chapter 7, page 107, for description.

2. **Wall Slide**

   See page 152 for description.

## STRENGTH TRAINING

### BASIC MOVE
# Dead Lift

**SPECIAL FEATURES** | Trap bar

**TARGET** | Legs, lower back, core

**PURPOSE** | This move is very similar to the barbell version, only it moves the load a little farther back, working your target muscles from a different angle.

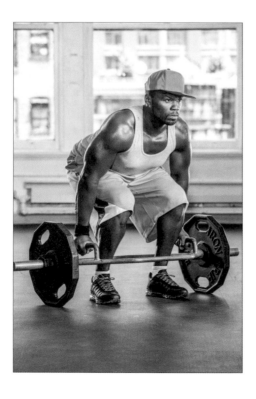 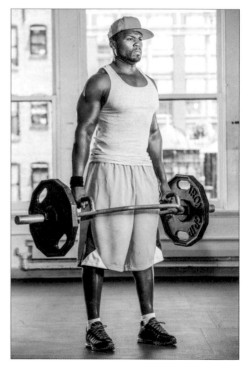

**GET READY** | Stand in the middle of a trap bar (also known as a hex bar) loaded with the appropriate weight. Place your feet no more than hip-width apart. Press your hips back and down, bending at the knees until you can take hold of the handles. Keep your chest up and your arms straight at your sides. Your thighs should be above parallel to the ground; your torso should be angled 45 degrees to the ground. Distribute your body weight evenly between your heels and the balls of your feet so that you're still able to wiggle your toes. Pull up slightly on the bar (with the bar still in contact with the ground). Think of this as "taking the slack" out of the bar.

**GO** | Holding your back tight, drive your heels into the ground. Contract your glutes and hamstrings while keeping your chest up and your back and core nice and tight. Push your hips forward and squeeze your glutes to finish the lift upright. Don't "squat" the weight as you rise; instead the bulk of your effort should come from pushing your hips forward. Reverse the motion by first pushing back your hips. When the bar reaches your knees, begin to bend them and lower your hips. Your chest should stay up, and your upper body should remain tight during the descent. Let the plates touch the ground. Then rest for a beat, making sure you're positioned properly before you begin the next rep. Avoid rounding your back. If you can no longer maintain proper back position, the set's a wrap.

**FIFTY SAYS** | "If you don't have a trap bar apparatus available at your gym, substitute dumbbells with your palms facing your body. This also shifts the weight back a bit compared to using a barbell for dead lifts."

**BASIC MOVE**
# Bench Press

See page 154 for description.

**BASIC MOVE**

# Hip Bridge

**SPECIAL FEATURES** | Single leg

**TARGET** | Hamstrings, glutes, stabilizers, core, lower back

**PURPOSE** | This body-weight move requires strength and stability. As a result, it improves core strength for other weight-training exercises and sports performance.

**GET READY** | Lie on your back and extend your arms so that they're 45 degrees (or a little more) from your body with your palms up. Bend your legs and bring your heels toward your butt. Keep your right heel in contact with the ground as you raise the toes of your right foot. Extend your left leg into the air until it's straight, making sure that both your upper legs create the same angle with the ground. Flex your left foot, pulling your toes toward your shin. Hold your left leg and foot in that position throughout the set.

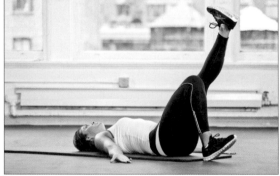

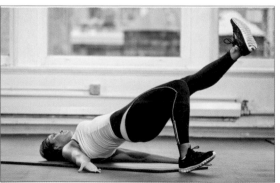

**GO** | Initiate the movement by driving your right heel into the ground, lifting your butt off the ground by contracting your glutes and hamstrings. Press your hips up until your body forms a straight line from your shoulders to your hips to your left ankle. Keep your back flat and your left leg straight throughout the set. Pull your abs into your midsection, keeping them tight throughout. Hold the contraction at the top and then slowly lower your body to the floor under control. Perform all reps on this side before switching to the other.

**FIFTY SAYS** | "Keep your upper legs in line throughout the set. It cheats the move if you drop your raised leg lower than your working leg and then lift at the top of the movement."

# Chin-Up

**SPECIAL FEATURES** | Shoulder-width grip, supinated

**TARGET** | Lower lats, smaller muscles of the upper back

**PURPOSE** | This variation provides more of a stretch in your lats, involving them in ways that other pull-ups or chin moves don't. It also allows for a deep contraction and longer hold at the top.

**GET READY** | Grasp a chin-up bar with a supinated grip (your palms facing toward your body), hands about shoulder-width apart. Let your body hang with your arms straight.

**GO** | Draw together your shoulder blades and lean back a bit as you begin to raise your body to the bar. Keep your shoulders down and your neck relaxed throughout the set. As your chin rises above the bar, force a deep contraction into your back by thinking it and feeling it. Slowly lower yourself back to the starting position, again feeling that stretch in your lower back.

**FIFTY SAYS** | "When you pull your shoulders back and down, and your chest forward, this move allows you to contract your back muscles with a vengeance. This is a serious exercise for bringing out detail in the small muscles of your upper back."

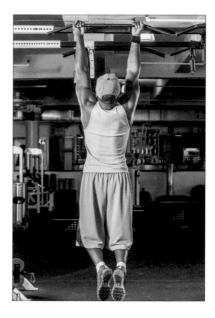

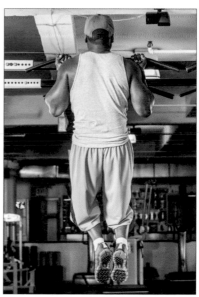

**BASIC MOVE**

# Prowler Push

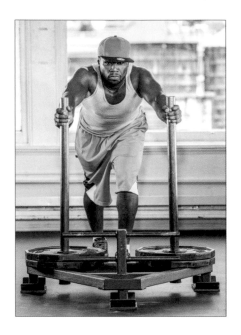

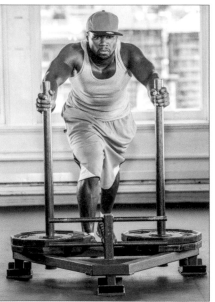

**SPECIAL FEATURES** | High hand position, upright

**TARGET** | Legs, glutes, sports performance

**PURPOSE** | This move integrates intense muscle contractions with muscular endurance, leading to more strength, more muscle, and better performance.

**GET READY** | Stand behind the prowler. Grip the vertical poles, placing your hands as high as you can while maintaining a full grasp. Hold your chest up and stand with one foot near the apparatus and the other 3 to 4 feet behind your front foot. Your lower body should be in a lunge position.

**GO** | Keeping your arms straight and chest up, press the prowler forward by driving through the ball of your front foot until your front leg and hip are fully extended. Next, bring your trailing leg forward, stepping beyond your front leg. Dig into the ground with your new front foot. As you continue pushing the prowler forward, keep your stepping pattern and upper body in sync so the prowler keeps advancing at a steady pace. Keep your arms straight and chest up as you push.

**FIFTY SAYS** | "Perform this move for distance instead of time so that you don't reward yourself for not working hard enough. You gotta keep at it until you've crossed the finish line, even if it feels like you just went a full round with Floyd."

# Hammer Curl

**SPECIAL FEATURES** | Dumbbell, seated

**TARGET** | Biceps, brachialis

**PURPOSE** | Underneath the two heads of your biceps lie the brachialis, the muscles that separate biceps from triceps. While the brachialis is barely visible unless developed, it can push your biceps up, making them look fuller and more detailed.

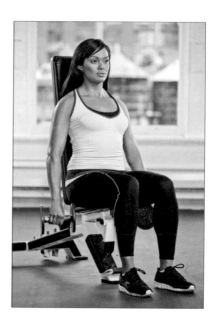

**GET READY** | Set an incline bench so that the back pad is tilted slightly back. Grasp a dumbbell in each hand and sit down, keeping your feet flat on the floor. Lie back on the bench, letting your arms hang at your sides, perpendicular to the ground, with your palms facing each other.

**GO** | Curl both dumbbells at once, keeping your palms facing each other and your elbows back. Your upper arms should remain perpendicular to the ground throughout the set. Squeeze your biceps at the peak. Lower the dumbbells with control until your arms are fully extended, palms still facing each other. Feel a stretch on the outside of your biceps.

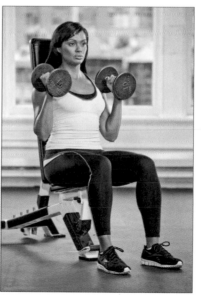

**FIFTY SAYS** | "It's hammer time! This move adds detail to the outside of your biceps—and to the inside middle of your arms, if you're able to achieve complete brachialis development."

## BASIC MOVE
# Triceps Extension

**SPECIAL FEATURES** | Dumbbell, supine, 10-degree decline

**TARGET** | Triceps

**PURPOSE** | This single-joint move isolates the triceps, allowing you to focus on enhancing detail and mass in this muscle group.

**GET READY** | Set a bench to a slight decline—you may need to place a box under one end if the benches at your gym are not adjustable (if you use a box, make sure the bench is secure). Lie back, holding a pair of dumbbells. Extend your arms fully with the dumbbells over your shoulders. Your upper arms should be perpendicular to the

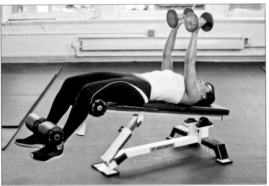

bench, slightly angled with the floor to create a greater stretch on your triceps throughout the set.

**GO** | Keeping your upper arms stationary, lower the dumbbells by bending your elbows, allowing the dumbbells to travel down until they are on either side of your head and your forearms are slightly below parallel to the ground (virtually parallel with the bench). Feel a stretch in your triceps. Squeeze your triceps to lift the weight back to the starting position, where your arms are fully extended.

**FIFTY SAYS** | "The slight decline of this move really activates your triceps. I feel much more action in my triceps than I do with the flat-bench version of this move, especially in the part of that muscle group up near my shoulder joint."

# Reverse Crunch

**SPECIAL FEATURES** | TRX suspension training straps

**TARGET** | Core, obliques, lower abs

**PURPOSE** | This move allows you to stretch and flex your rectus abdominis (your six-pack); it also involves stabilizers and side abs, especially your obliques.

**GET READY** | Attach a TRX to a high anchor position and adjust the straps so the handles are close to knee level when you're standing. Place one foot at a time in each of the TRX flexible foot cradles (below the more rigid handles). Get into the straps in the most comfortable way for you—it's a little tricky at first. Place your hands on the ground and facedown. Extend your body so that you're in a plank position with your body straight from ankles to head. Your arms should be fully extended and perpendicular to the ground, with your hands directly under your shoulders. Your feet should be suspended directly below the anchor point of the TRX straps so that they are perpendicular to the ground. Before you begin the move, make sure that your core is engaged and your back is tight.

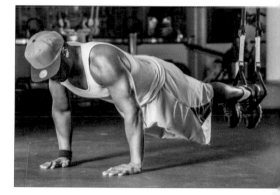

**GO** | Initiate the movement by contracting your core and raising your hips so that your body forms a pike. Once your hips are elevated, bend your knees and bring them toward your chest. Make sure to keep your feet together, and your quads and hips tight as your knees move in toward your upper body. Your back will round slightly, and that's fine for

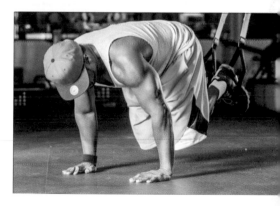

this move. Pull your lower body into your chest until your knees are as tight to your chest as your range of motion comfortably allows. Reverse the motion by slowly extending your knees out from under your hips until your legs are straight and you are in a pike position. Next, lower your hips with control, coming to a rest when your body reaches the plank position. Keep your core engaged, arms straight, and the rest of your body tight throughout the set.

**FIFTY SAYS** | "This is a great move for crunching your abs from the opposite direction from most abs moves. Just make sure that you don't allow your hips to sag or use momentum to bring your knees into your chest. Keep the move controlled and deliberate, and really crunch down on your abs."

## STRENGTH 4-B

### Dynamic Warm-Up/Flexibility

| Exercise | Sets | Reps | Load | Tempo | Rest | Intensity |
|---|---|---|---|---|---|---|
| Side-Lying Spinal Twist | 1 | 5/side | Body-weight | Moderate | None | Low |
| Hip Flexor Stretch | 1 | 5/side | Body-weight | Moderate | None | Low |
| Twisting Lunge Stretch | 1 | 5/side | Body-weight | Moderate | None | Low |
| Drop Step Lunge | 1 | 5/side | Body-weight | Moderate | None | Low |

### Activation Drills

| Drill | Sets | Reps | Load | Tempo[1] | Rest | Intensity |
|---|---|---|---|---|---|---|
| Lateral Walk | 1 | 10–12/side | Body-weight | 2011 | None | Low |
| Wall Slide | 1 | 10 | Body-weight | 2011 | None | Low |

### Strength Training

| Exercise | Sets[2] | Reps | Load[3] | Tempo[1] | Rest (secs) | Intensity |
|---|---|---|---|---|---|---|
| A1. Front Squat | 3–4 | 8–10 | TBD | 3010 | 30, 20, 10 | High |
| A2. Inverted Row | 3–4 | 8–10 | TBD | 3010 | 30, 20, 10 | High |
| A3. Hip Bridge/Leg Curl | 3–4 | 8–10 | TBD | 3010 | 30, 20, 10 | High |
| A4. Rope Pull | 3–4 | 150 feet | TBD | 3010 | 30, 20, 10 | High |
| A5. Biceps Curl/Press | 3–4 | 8–10 | TBD | 2020 | 30, 20, 10 | High |
| A6. Box Shuffle | 3–4 | 30 seconds | Body-Weight | Fast | 30, 20, 10 | High |
| A7. Triceps Extension | 3–4 | 8–10 | TBD | 3010 | 30, 20, 10 | High |
| A8. Core Press | 3–4 | 30 seconds | Body-Weight | Hold | 120 | High |

[1] "Tempo" refers to the speed of movement. For example, 3-1-1-0 means: 3 seconds lowering the weight; 1 second pause in the lengthened position; 1 second to raise the weight; no pause ("0") in the contracted position.

[2] Perform each exercise, all 8 of 'em, in succession, resting 30 seconds between each one, at least during Week 10. At the end of A8 (the core press), rest 120 seconds. You'll need it. Then repeat the circuit again under the same scenario, until you've completed 3 circuits—4 only if you can handle it.

During Week 11, decrease your rest in between moves to 20 seconds while keeping the 120-second break at the end of each circuit. During Week 12, decrease it to 10 seconds—barely time to suck down a few gulps of air.

[3] Choose a weight at which you fail in the desired rep range. For the bench press, if you can do only 7 reps, your weight is too heavy. If you can do 11, it's too light. Adjust your weight selection accordingly.

**Flexibility training:** Perform immediately post-workout. See Chapter 6, page 61, for details.

**Foam rolling:** Perform immediately after stretching. See Chapter 6, page 72, for details.

## DYNAMIC WARM-UP/FLEXIBILITY

1. **Side-Lying Spinal Twist**

   See Chapter 7, page 88, for description.

2. **Hip Flexor Stretch**

   See Chapter 7, page 90, for description.

3. **Twisting Lunge Stretch**

   See Chapter 7, page 105, for description.

4. **Drop Step Lunge**

   See page 174 for description.

## ACTIVATION DRILLS

1. **Lateral Walk**

   See Chapter 7, page 107, for description.

2. **Wall Slide**

   See page 152 for description.

## STRENGTH TRAINING

### BASIC MOVE
# Front Squat

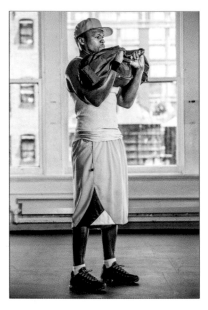

**SPECIAL FEATURES** | Sandbag

**TARGET** | Legs, upper body, stabilizers, core

**PURPOSE** | This move takes you through the same range of motion as other squat moves, albeit with a shifting weight load.

**GET READY** | Hold a sandbag on the front of your shoulders by wrapping your arms underneath it, keeping your upper arms as upright as you can throughout the set. Stand tall with your feet slightly wider than your hips. Tighten your core, pull your chest up, and point your elbows straight ahead.

**GO** | Maintaining the weight on the back half of your feet, move your hips down and back, descending into a squat. As you move downward, focus on keeping your elbows high. Squat as deeply as you can while keeping good form, allowing your upper legs to go below parallel if possible. Reverse the motion by driving through your feet and extending your knees and hips. Reset at the top and repeat for reps.

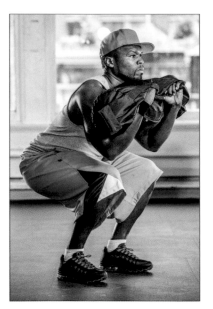

**FIFTY SAYS** | "This variation is great for getting you accustomed to handling an unwieldy load. It's like squatting with a really heavy bag of groceries."

# Inverted Row

**SPECIAL FEATURES** | Pronated grip

**TARGET** | Lats, smaller muscles of your upper back, core

**PURPOSE** | This rowing/pull-up variation works your back through a different range of motion than other moves in the Formula 50 workout do.

**GET READY** | Take hold of a Smith Machine or squat rack bar with an overhand grip, hands slightly wider than your shoulders. Walk your feet forward 3 to 4 feet until you're hanging underneath the bar. Extend your arms and lower your body, digging your heels into the floor so that your body forms a straight line from ankles to head.

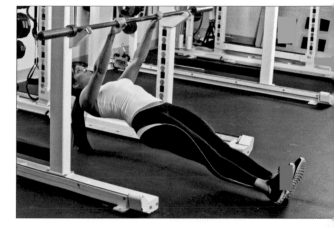

**GO** | While keeping your body tight and in line from ankles to head, tuck your chin back, pull your shoulders down, and pull your body up to the bar. Try to touch the bar with your chest, feeling a contraction in your upper back. Reverse the motion by slowly lowering your body, keeping your chest up, body straight, and shoulders back and down. Emphasize a stretch in the muscles of your back, lowering your body until your arms are straight.

**FIFTY SAYS** | "You can also place your heels on a bench to elevate your body so that you're parallel to the ground at the beginning. This changes the angle and increases the amount of weight you're lifting for each rep."

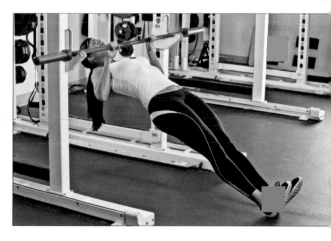

# Hip Bridge/Leg Curl

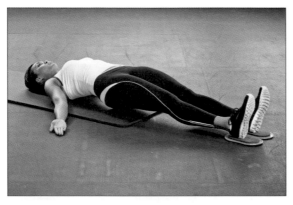

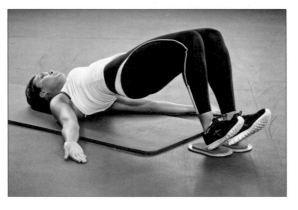

**SPECIAL FEATURES** | Body weight, sliding pads

**TARGET** | Abs, glutes, lower back

**PURPOSE** | This move combines deep contractions of your backside and abs through a unique range of motion.

**GET READY** | Lie on a fixed pad, legs fully extended, arms out to your sides at an angle. Press your heels into two sliding pads, and hold your body tight.

**GO** | Begin to pull your feet toward your hips as you raise your hips off the ground, holding a contraction in your glutes throughout the set. Arch your back and press your hips up as high as you comfortably can. Avoid using momentum or the "slide" to increase your range of motion. Hold the upper position for a couple of seconds, then reverse the motion. Press your feet back out slowly and, with control, gently place your hips back on the ground.

**FIFTY SAYS** | "You work your abs and glutes in a lot of the exercises during Formula 50, but this move is great because the stretch position for the abs is more challenging than the contraction."

# Rope Pull

**SPECIAL FEATURES** | Sled

**TARGET** | Legs, core, arms, back

**PURPOSE** | This whole-body move primarily works your back.

**GET READY** | Attach a long rope to a sled that's been loaded with the appropriate amount of weight for you. Take hold of the other end of the rope and move away from the sled until the rope has no slack. Face the sled, and lower your body into a quarter squat, thighs above parallel to the ground. Press your hips back, and hold your chest up and shoulders down.

**GO** | Move the sled toward you by pulling on the rope, rowing the weight. As you pull with one arm, place your opposite hand on the rope 2 feet or so beyond your work-ing hand, closer to the sled. Keep the sled moving, switch-ing arms in a rhythm that allows for continual motion. Maintain the integrity of your body position throughout the set. Don't let your upper body lean too far forward or back. Also, don't rotate your torso excessively as you reach out with your arms. Keep your lower body tight and your core strong as you use the muscles of your back to bring the sled toward your body. Allow the excess rope to fall between your legs. Cover your target distances with as many lengths of rope as it takes (for instance, if you have a 30-foot rope and your goal is 60 feet per set, then perform 2 full rounds before resting).

**FIFTY SAYS** | "This exercise is designed to work your back, but it may leave your whole body shaking. I love this one."

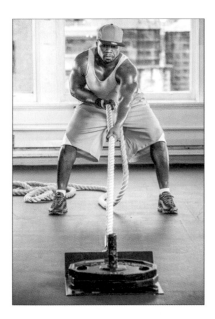

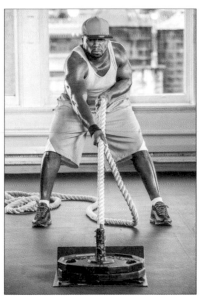

**BASIC MOVE**

# Biceps Curl/Press

**SPECIAL FEATURES** | Dumbbell, seated 90-degree angle

**TARGET** | Biceps, shoulders

**PURPOSE** | This move not only works your biceps and shoulders but also integrates transitional muscles as you rotate your shoulders to switch from curling to pressing.

**GET READY** | Sit on a bench with a back support in the upright position, as close to 90 degrees as the bench allows. Hold a dumbbell in each hand with your palms facing forward.

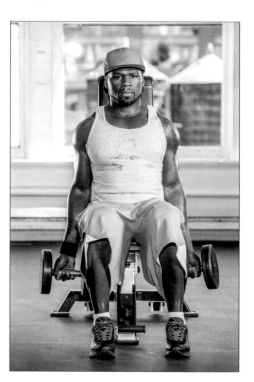 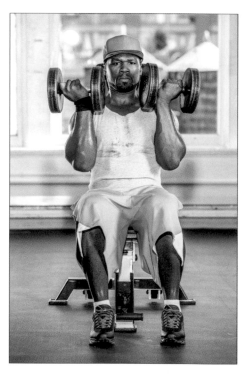

**GO** | Keeping your elbows in line with your body, curl both dumbbells up to your shoulders. Emphasize a contraction in your biceps, and then rotate your palms so that they face away from your body. Now press the weights above your head until your arms are straight but your elbows are not locked. Make sure to keep a space between your shoulders and ears so that your shoulders actively engage with the weight at the top of the move. Contract your delts, then slowly lower the dumbbells, feeling a stretch in your shoulders. Rotate your palms so that they're facing your body at the bottom of the shoulder press. Then, extend your arms with control to return to the starting position, feeling a stretch in your biceps.

**FIFTY SAYS** | "Transitional moves not only help you develop muscularity for more than one body part, but they teach your body how to adapt to real-world moves that require explosiveness."

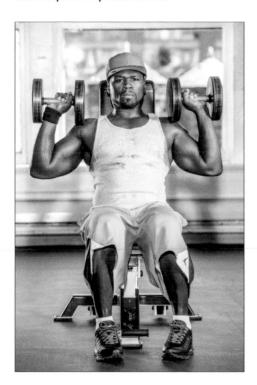 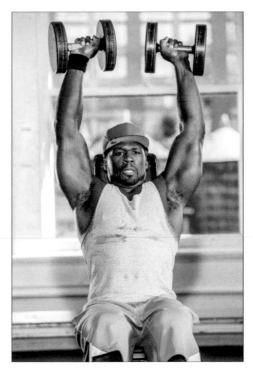

BASIC MOVE
## BASIC MOVE
# Box Shuffle

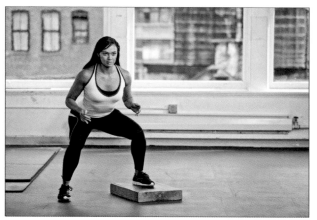

**SPECIAL FEATURES** | A 3- to 6-inch box

**TARGET** | Cardio, legs

**PURPOSE** | To increase heart and metabolic rate for increased fat burning.

**GET READY** | Set up a low box, about 3 to 6 inches tall. Place one foot on the box and hold most of your weight on the other foot on the ground. Your feet should be about a yard apart. Keep your chest up and your knees slightly bent.

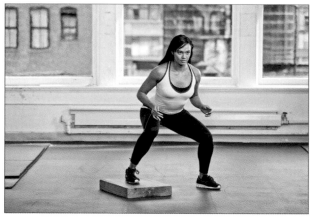

**GO** | Shuffle laterally across the box. When your foot touches the floor on the other side, decelerate by planting that foot on the ground, absorbing the impact with your hips. (You should mirror the starting position at this point.) Quickly reverse directions and shuffle laterally back to the side you started on. Decelerate with your other foot and hip this time. Over and back counts as one rep. Keep shuffling side-to-side for the given number of reps, maintaining an athletic position without sacrificing form for speed.

**FIFTY SAYS** | "This is the kind of move you might see defensive backs doing in football practice. It never hurts to be fast on your feet—in the gym or in life."

# Triceps Extension

**SPECIAL FEATURES** | Standing, TRX straps

**TARGET** | Triceps, core

**PURPOSE** | This move works your triceps in a different way, requiring you to hold your body tight to emphasize your target muscles.

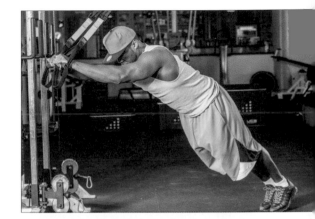

**GET READY** | Attach two TRX straps to a high anchor and adjust the straps so that they're about 6 feet long. Face away from the anchor point and take hold of the handles, with your palms facing away from your body. Take a step or two forward and then extend your arms in front of you until the TRX becomes taught. Your palms should face the floor and your arms should be roughly parallel to the floor. Keeping your arms straight, lean into the straps so that they support your body weight. Your body should make about a 60-degree angle with the ground. Make sure your body forms one line from ankles to head and that your core is tight and shoulders are down.

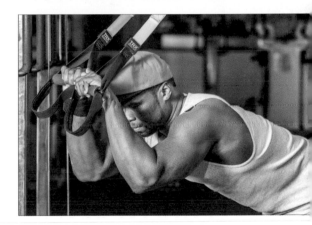

**GO** | Initiate the movement by bending at your elbows, letting your forearms move back as your body descends. Allow your hands to move toward your head, but make sure that your upper arms stay still. Feel a stretch in your triceps as your hands get close to your head. Reverse the motion by contracting your triceps as you straighten your arms to return to the starting position. Make sure to keep your elbows in place, your body in one line, and your core tight throughout.

**FIFTY SAYS** | "You can adjust the difficulty of this move by shifting your foot position. The closer your feet are to the anchor point—and the smaller the angle your body makes with the ground—the more difficult the exercise is."

**BASIC MOVE**

# Core Press

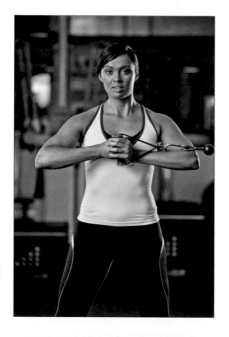

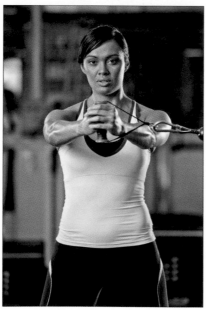

**SPECIAL FEATURES** | Cable or resistance band

**TARGET** | Core

**PURPOSE** | To develop strength and definition in your midsection for better appearance and athletic performance.

**GET READY** | Set up a cable pulley or anchor a resistance band at chest height. Grab the handle with a hand-over-hand grip, facing perpendicular to the line of the cable or band. Take a step or two away from the anchor point until you feel tension in the cable. Place your feet hip-distance apart and hold your chest up, shoulders down, and core tight, with your hands close to your chest.

**GO** | Press the handle away from your body, extending your arms, keeping them parallel to the ground at chest height. Pause for a second, then pull your hands back to your chest, maintaining control throughout. Complete all reps on one side, then switch to the other.

**FIFTY SAYS** | "What's great about this move is how much you feel it working the side of your abs closer to the cable machine."

## STRENGTH 4-C

### Dynamic Warm-Up/Flexibility

| Exercise | Sets | Reps | Load | Tempo | Rest | Intensity |
|---|---|---|---|---|---|---|
| Side-Lying Spinal Twist | 1 | 5/side | Body-weight | Moderate | None | Low |
| Hip Flexor Stretch | 1 | 5/side | Body-weight | Moderate | None | Low |
| Twisting Lunge Stretch | 1 | 5/side | Body-weight | Moderate | None | Low |
| Drop Step Lunge | 1 | 5/side | Body-weight | Moderate | None | Low |

### Activation Drills

| Drill | Sets | Reps | Load | Tempo[1] | Rest | Intensity |
|---|---|---|---|---|---|---|
| Lateral Walk | 1 | 10–12/side | Body-weight | 2011 | None | Low |
| Wall Slide | 1 | 10 | Body-weight | 2011 | None | Low |

### Strength Training

| Exercise | Sets[2] | Reps | Load[3] | Tempo[1] | Rest (secs) | |
|---|---|---|---|---|---|---|
| A1. Lunge | 3–4 | 8–10/side | TBD | 2010 | 30, 20, 10 | High |
| A2. Bench Press | 3–4 | 8–10 | TBD | 3010 | 30, 20, 10 | High |
| A3. Glute-Ham Raise | 3–4 | 8–10 | TBD | 2010 | 30, 20, 10 | High |
| A4. Farmer's Walk | 3–4 | 150 feet | TBD | Moderate | 30, 20, 10 | High |
| A5. Shoulder Press | 3–4 | 8–10 | TBD | 20X0 | 30, 20, 10 | High |
| A6. Zottman Curl | 3–4 | 8–10 | TBD | 2020 | 30, 20, 10 | High |
| A7. High Row | 3–4 | 8–10 | TBD | 3010 | 30, 20, 10 | High |
| A8. Medicine Ball Slam | 3–4 | 10–12 | TBD | Hold | 120 | High |

[1] "Tempo" refers to the speed of movement. For example, 3-1-1-0 means: 3 seconds lowering the weight; 1 second pause in the lengthened position; 1 second to raise the weight; no pause ("0") in the contracted position.

[2] Perform each exercise, all 8 of 'em, in succession, resting 30 seconds between each one, at least during Week 10. At the end of A8 (the medicine ball slam), rest 120 seconds. You'll need it. Then repeat the circuit again under the same scenario, until you've completed 3 circuits—4 only if you can handle it.

During Week 11, decrease your rest in between moves to 20 seconds while keeping the 120-second break at the end of each circuit. During Week 12, decrease rest between moves to 10 seconds—barely time to suck down a few gulps of air.

[3] Choose a weight at which you fail in the desired rep range. For the bench press, if you can do only 7 reps, your weight is too heavy. If you can do 11, it's too light. Adjust your weight selection accordingly.

**Flexibility training:** Perform immediately post-workout. See Chapter 6, page 61, for details.

**Foam rolling:** Perform immediately after stretching. See Chapter 6, page 72, for details.

## DYNAMIC WARM-UP/FLEXIBILITY

1. **Side-Lying Spinal Twist**

   See Chapter 7, page 88, for description.

2. **Hip Flexor Stretch**

   See Chapter 7, page 90, for description.

3. **Twisting Lunge Stretch**

   See Chapter 7, page 105, for description.

4. **Drop Step Lunge**

   See page 174 for description.

## ACTIVATION DRILLS

1. **Lateral Walk**

   See Chapter 7, page 107, for description.

2. **Wall Slide**

   See page 152 for description.

## STRENGTH TRAINING

**BASIC MOVE**

# Lunge

**SPECIAL FEATURES** | Bulgarian style, split legs, dumbbells

**TARGET** | Legs, glutes, core

**PURPOSE** | This lunge variation requires more balance and muscular effort from your front leg.

**GET READY** | Hold a pair of dumbbells and face away from a bench. Carefully place one foot behind you on top of the bench. Hold the other leg straight and slightly in front of you, standing upright with the dumbbells at your sides. Make sure that your torso is upright, your chest is up, and shoulders are down.

**GO** | Slowly drop your back knee toward the floor. Bend your front leg at the knee and hips, letting your upper body travel straight down. Keep your torso upright throughout, preventing it from leaning forward as you descend. Feel a stretch across the top of your front leg, then reverse the motion by driving forcefully through your front foot until you return to the starting position. Try to avoid pushing against the bench with your rear foot, as that undercuts the work your front leg must perform. Complete all reps on one side, then switch to the other.

**FIFTY SAYS** | "Your back leg is really just there to spot you. All the effort comes from your front leg."

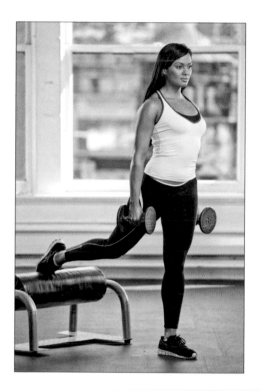
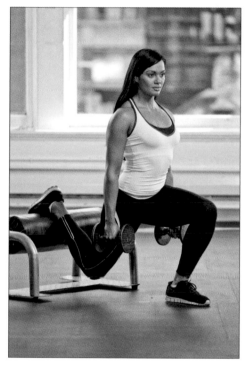

## BASIC MOVE

# Bench Press

See page 154 for description.

# Glute-Ham Raise

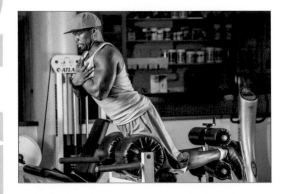

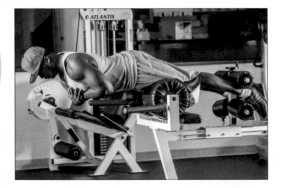

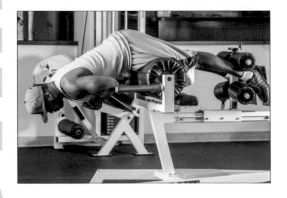

**SPECIAL FEATURES** | Standard

**TARGET** | Glutes, hamstrings, core

**PURPOSE** | A glutes-ham machine allows you to bend your knees in the middle of the exercise, involving more hamstrings movement than regular hyperextensions.

**GET READY** | Set up a glutes-ham machine so that your knees are directly on, or immediately behind, the pad. Secure the backs of your ankles under the pads. At the start, your knees should be bent, torso upright, chest up, and arms crossed over your chest. Before beginning the movement, engage your glutes, hamstrings, and core.

**GO** | While keeping your back flat, lower your upper body toward the floor as you straighten your legs. At the bottom of the movement, your upper body should be below parallel to the ground and your legs should be straight. Don't allow your lower back to round; hold the natural curve in your lower back throughout the set. Contract your glutes and pull with your hamstrings to raise your upper body. As you pass parallel, bend your knees until you return to the starting position. Keep your back flat throughout the set.

**FIFTY SAYS** | "If your gym doesn't have a glutes-ham machine, then substitute hyperextensions for this move. The action is a bit different, but hyperextensions also work the glutes and hamstrings."

# Farmer's Walk

**SPECIAL FEATURES** | Dumbbells

**TARGET** | Core, grip, forearms, overall muscular endurance

**PURPOSE** | This move primarily targets your forearms and grip, but it's also great for increasing muscular endurance for enhanced athletic performance.

**GET READY** | Grab a pair of heavy dumbbells and hold them at your sides with your palms facing each other. Stand with your chest up and your shoulders down and back. Your feet should be about hip-width apart.

**GO** | Holding the dumbbells with a firm grip so that you don't drop them, begin walking. Make sure that your core is tight with your upper body upright. Complete the prescribed distance. If you need to change directions during the set, rotate slowly so that you minimize the strain on your spine.

**FIFTY SAYS** | "While you'll feel this move mostly in your grip, it's important you maintain good posture throughout the set."

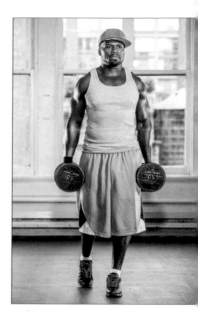

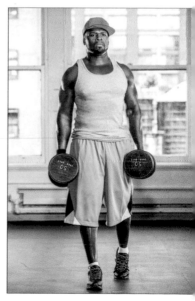

## BASIC MOVE
# Shoulder Press

**SPECIAL FEATURES** | Barbell, push-press

**TARGET** | Shoulders, core, whole body

**PURPOSE** | This move directly targets the shoulders, but the push-press element brings in much of the rest of your body, including core and legs.

**GET READY** | Load a barbell with appropriate weights. Grasp it with your hands slightly wider than your shoulders. Unrack the barbell and hold it at your shoulders. (You can set it up at this height, or you set it up lower and "clean" it into place.) Your palms should be facing away from your body. Hold your chest up and core tight, and stand with your feet about hip-width apart.

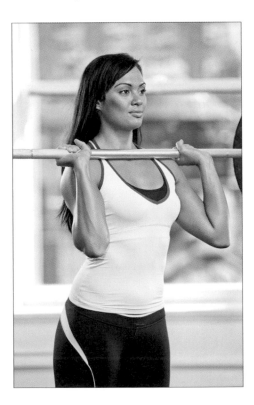 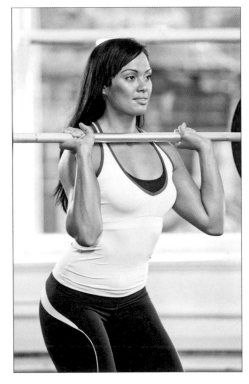

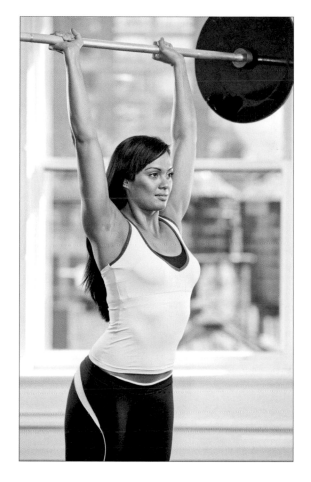

**GO** | Bend your knees a bit while keeping your chest up. Next, drive explosively through your legs, using the power of your lower body to help push the barbell over your head. Press the bar up until your arms are fully extended and you are standing upright. Stabilize your body and the weight at the top of the motion, then bend your elbows, slowly returning the weight to shoulder level, keeping your legs straight. Make sure you are in the proper starting position before beginning the next rep.

**FIFTY SAYS** | "You get a lot of power by bending your knees and integrating your lower body into the pressing movement. Just make sure you keep your core tight and your form proper to avoid injury."

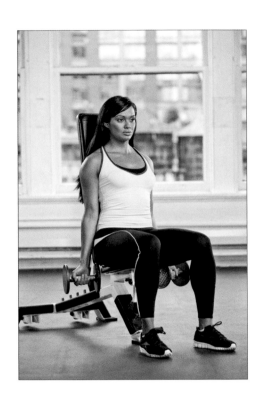
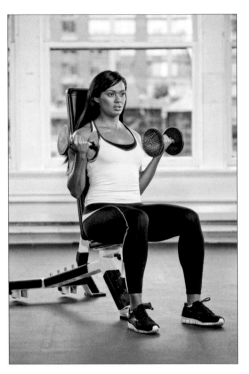

**BASIC MOVE**

# Zottman Curl

**SPECIAL FEATURES** | Dumbbell, seated, 90-degree angle

**TARGET** | Biceps, forearms, brachialis

**PURPOSE** | This version of biceps curls recruits your forearms and brachialis more than the pronated version does.

**GET READY** | Set up a seated bench so the backrest is nearly vertical. Sit on the bench and hold a pair of dumbbells at your sides. Turn your palms so they face forward.

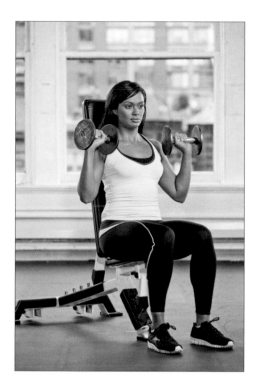
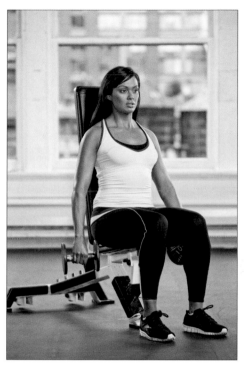

**GO** | Curl the dumbbells to your shoulders, keeping your elbows still at your sides. At the top, rotate your wrists 180 degrees so that your palms face away from you. Lower the dumbbells with control, keeping your elbows still at your sides. When your arms are fully extended, rotate your wrists 180 degrees again, until they are in the starting position. Pause for a moment, then begin the next rep.

**FIFTY SAYS** | "Reversing the direction of your palms for lowering the weights really gets the muscles of your forearms to fire."

# High Row

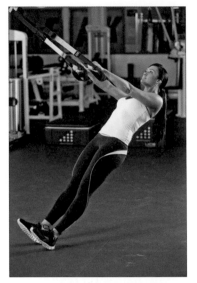

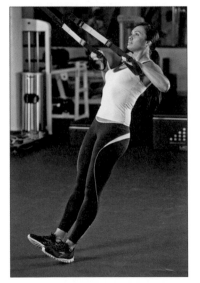

**SPECIAL FEATURES** | TRX, body weight

**TARGET** | Back, whole body

**PURPOSE** | This version of row not only works your lats but also requires stabilization throughout your entire body.

**GET READY** | Attach two TRX straps to a high, stable location. The straps should be 6 to 8 feet long, allowing you to adjust the difficulty level. Face the anchor point and step back 2 to 3 feet—the farther away from the anchor your feet are, the easier the exercise. Keeping your body straight from ankles to head, dig your heels into the ground, and lean back until your arms are straight. Your body should be angled at about a 45-degree angle with the ground. Hold your chest up and your shoulders back and down, making sure that you feel no strain in your neck.

**GO** | Pull your body up toward the TRX handles, bending your elbows. Keep your wrists straight, and your hands, elbows, and shoulders in line. Use the muscles of your upper back to pull your body high enough that your elbows are behind you. Emphasize a contraction in these upper-back muscles, holding that for a second. Slowly let your body angle back toward the ground, emphasizing a stretch in your back. Keep your chest up and shoulders down throughout. Maintain a straight line from ankles to head throughout the move.

**FIFTY SAYS** | "Regardless of your fitness level, you can make this a great exercise by adjusting your foot position; just make sure that you hold your body straight, from ankles to head, at whatever angle of motion is appropriate for you."

204

# Medicine Ball Slam

**SPECIAL FEATURES** | Standard

**TARGET** | Shoulders, muscular endurance, core

**PURPOSE** | This move not only helps open your shoulders but also works your core and lower body.

**GET READY** | Grab a medicine ball with both hands, palms facing each other. Stand with your feet about shoulder-width apart. Raise the medicine ball above and slightly behind your head. Your arms should be close to fully extended at the top.

**GO** | Initiate the movement by explosively throwing the medicine ball onto the floor. Think about forcefully contracting your core to assist the motion. Be careful that the ball does not come back to hit you after you throw it (depending on how much it weighs, it may bounce). Squat down, pick up the medicine ball, and push back up to standing, raising it above your head with straight arms. Reset your feet if necessary and continue, completing the desired number of reps.

**FIFTY SAYS** | "These might sound easy enough, but after you perform a few reps, you really start to feel this exercise working."

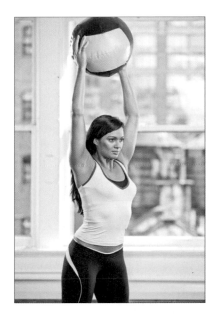

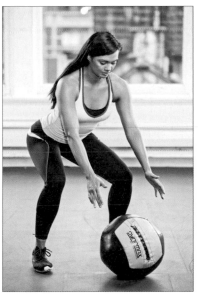

# 10

# FAQs That Will Arise During Formula 50

**Q** **I'm starting from scratch here. Can I really do this program?**

**A** If I set my mind to anything, I think I can do it. I had to build that confidence over time and with success; I can legitimately say that because of how far I've come in my life. Tell me you made a million dollars when you already had a million dollars, and I'll say, "So what!" Tell me you had nothing and then became a millionaire, and I'll say, "Okay, you did something." Same with fitness: I'll be the most impressed by those of you with the courage to start from scratch.

The hardest part for you will be getting started. No getting around it. But if you stick with this program, you'll reach a point where anything will seem possible fitness-wise. A triathlon or bodybuilding show will seem less hard than entering a gym for the first time seems now. Formula 50 takes you through this challenging beginner's stage.

**Q** **How important is it to find and follow fitness role models as I embark upon Formula 50?**

**A** Role models are important, whether they're positive or negative. I'll give you an example. The heroes of my youth were drug dealers. Sounds foolish or even stupid, right? They were my heroes because I didn't know any better, and because they had this rebel energy. They led intense crews in the darkness. Today, though, if those same guys tell me a story about how it was back then, I always look to see if there's a gold tooth in their mouth. I'm thinking, *Let's see now, maybe they got ONE thing to show for that time period.* To become one of their followers? Nine times out of ten, you ended up dead or in jail. I'm an exception.

The same goes for health and fitness. If you model your behavior on people who are overweight and don't exercise, you'll end up dead or with type 2 diabetes (and then dead, after an amputation or two). So follow those who set positive examples. Follow me. Follow Arnold or The Rock. Follow the guy at the office who carries around his chicken and broccoli in Tupperware. Follow all of us. Don't leave any stones unturned in your search for health and wellness.

Don't forget who helped you either. I hate that. Once you look and feel like a new man or woman, don't be ungrateful or blinded by that success or your new image. Always remember: *How did I get here?* When I arrive someplace, I'm going to remember if I took a cab or walked.

**Q** **You talk so much about the importance of breakfast, and the meal plans contain examples. What's an ideal breakfast for me to be eating on the Formula 50 plan?**

**A** The ideal breakfast doesn't come in a box with a cartoon character on the front. It includes protein, some healthy fat, a moderate number of complex carbs, and a healthy dose of fiber along with those carbs. Eggs and a bowl of oatmeal with blueberries would be a real breakfast of champions. So would cottage cheese with walnuts and strawberries on top. So would all the breakfasts in the Formula 50 meal plans.

Don't be afraid of eggs, yoke and all. They're not going to hurt you. Only remove the yolk if you want to cut some calories; otherwise, they contain important nutrients. Swapping out two whole eggs and replacing them with five egg whites can save you 65 calories and 9 grams of fat. That's 455 fewer calories in 1 week, so nothing to sneeze at.

Breakfasts consisting only of carbs are the worst, especially when those carbs are simple sugars. That approach sets you up for a blood sugar crash that'll leave you wishing that 11:30 am meeting was nap time instead.

**Q You hype fiber a lot in this book. What's the big deal?**

**A** Fiber does at least three things that are extremely important: It makes you feel full, it keeps your blood sugar stable rather than crazy, and it helps "scrub" your digestive systems of toxins, a function that could help prevent cancer over time. While it's technically a carb, fiber is more like protein when it comes to the amount of energy the body must invest attempting to digest it. Unfortunately, the average American consumes about half the recommended amount of fiber. Blame it on too much fast food and not enough fiber-rich fruits and vegetables.

**Q So what's a simple way to add more fiber to my diet?**

**A** The Formula 50 meal plans are designed to ensure that you consume enough fiber each day. Beyond that, make sure you eat plenty of vegetables. At breakfast, throw some chopped mushrooms and broccoli into your omelet, for example. For snacks, include chopped veggies like cauliflower and celery. If celery sounds boring, load it with some tuna fish or natural peanut butter. At dinner, steam vegetables to accompany your protein source.

**Q Why do I always want comfort foods? Why are they so hard to resist?**

**A** Many people look at food as a reward or a comfort or a way to bring them back to their childhood. There are so many emotions attached to different kinds of eating, and if you come to terms with those emotions, it becomes much easier to lose weight. I'm not saying you have to detach yourself from emotions and food; the connection to memories and places is part of being human. But when you're eating fried chicken and

French fries and coleslaw and double portions of everything because *that's what we used to eat on family weekend picnics*, your emotions are getting the best of you where food is concerned.

**Q How do I juggle fitness with the rest of my life? That's always my downfall.**

**A** I'm ambitious, and my ambition is like an endless tunnel. Running through it sometimes gives me tunnel vision. I see what I want to achieve and I race after it until I cross that finish line (or die tryin'). That can be good, but it can also lead you to neglect other important things in your life. For example, you can fail to make spending time with your kids a priority. I watched Em [Eminem] go through that. Eventually he slowed down from his touring because he wanted to see his daughter, Hailie. He didn't want to come home one day and see a full-grown woman he didn't even know. His example made me more aware and conscious of the need for balance because he was ahead of me in his career. I lost my mom when I was 8 years old and was hustling by the time I was 12, so I always want to be there for my son.

This lesson also relates very much to fitness and working out. Training and eating right can help you stay balanced, so keep them in perspective and integrate them into your lifestyle. Don't let your life crowd out fitness, and don't let fitness take over your life. Either way, you got it wrong.

**Q Can I deviate even slightly from the meal plans in Formula 50, or will that mess me up?**

**A** The Formula 50 meal plans are guides. They're not as specific as NASA launch codes. As you progress through the program, you'll get to know your body better, and you can adapt and change based on how your body responds. That might seem like a large responsibility, but you should learn enough throughout this book to determine, "You know what, I don't like the way I feel after consuming carbs, so I'm going to tweak up my protein a little higher and tweak down my carbs."

Always stay true to the spirit of the meal plans and dietary advice, however. If you find that you consistently fall short of my plan's protein recommendation, for example, you've lost your way, nutritionally speaking. The exciting development will come when you can make meals based on, but different from, the ones offered in this book. At that point, the possibilities become nearly endless. You'll never be bored again in the kitchen, and you'll look like a million bucks. That's a win-win.

**Q** **What time of day should I work out? Will morning workouts produce better results than evening workouts or vice versa?**

**A** Not really. You're not going to burn more calories doing a workout at lunch than you would doing the same workout after dinner, assuming you put forth the same effort in both sessions. The best time of day to work out is the time when you will actually work out, and do so with the necessary intensity.

Especially when I'm touring, I like to get up and work out early. It gives me a chance to think about what I'm going to do the rest of the day. Jumping on the treadmill first thing jolts me like my morning coffee. Having done that, I feel better approaching everything else I have to do that day. It's cool.

If you can't answer that morning alarm with a workout, find the time of day or night when you can. Likewise, if your packed schedule compels you to train at 11 p.m., great—as long as you train effectively then. If you're shuffling around like a zombie on Xanax in the gym at that hour, that's not your time. Remember, Formula 50 is about making fitness part of your lifestyle. Train when it fits in with the rest of your life.

**Q** **I've read a lot of conflicting information about how much water I should drink. How much should I drink on your program, Fifty?**

**A** A lot. Probably more than you are now. Water constitutes up to 75 percent of the human body and influences virtually every body process—including building muscle and burning fat. So don't leave your body high and dry. The International Sports Sciences Association (ISSA) says to drink eight to twelve glasses of water a day. One trick is to just drink a glass every even or odd hour all day. If you're active—and if you're reading this book, you are, right?—ISSA would like for you to add an additional 16 ounces for every pound shed during exercise. A sure sign that you're not getting enough: if your urine looks dark yellow. If you see that, head straight from the bathroom to the kitchen sink and pour yourself a glass of $H_2O$.

**Q** **What about other beverages like coffee, tea, soda, and alcohol? What's okay and what isn't?**

**A** Research suggests that, drunk in moderation, coffee isn't harmful and may actually be healthy. Drink no more than three cups a day, though, and I definitely wouldn't add sugar, although a splash of milk or cream is fine. If you're dragging a bit before your workout, coffee can serve as a great pick-me-up. Like coffee, tea has healthy antioxidants and no downside if you don't add sugar. Drink up!

Sugary sodas are off-limits on my program. Diet variations are okay, although I wouldn't rely on them too heavily. Treat them as an occasional indulgence, rather than as a habit.

Alcohol can be drunk in moderation, meaning one or two drinks a day of light beer or wine. Hard liquor doesn't have a place on my program.

**Q** I've never seen some of the exercises in this program. What's wrong with the old standards?

**A** This program *is* filled with the old standards: compound barbell and dumbbell moves and body-weight exercises. What you won't see are a lot of newer exercises, like machine curls, that involve sitting down and moving one muscle at one joint. You sit all day; you really want to go to the gym to sit some more? Those are better than nothing but less than ideal. They don't build coordination and balance. They don't maximize caloric expenditure. They don't develop very much functional strength. They don't create the sort of hormonal response needed to burn fat and build muscle with maximum efficiency.

The exercises included here accomplish all those things and more. We've chosen them precisely because they work so well with metabolic resistance training. Once you're finished with the Formula 50 program, I'm confident you'll never want to sit on some dopey exercise machine again.

**Q** It seems like cooking is part of your meal plans, but I'm not very good at it. Any tips?

**A** Time to graduate from fast food and frozen dinners. You don't need to be the second coming of the Iron Chef. Just start with a few items or utensils, like a knife, a pan, a pot, and a rice cooker—you can cook rice or vegetables in there. Broil or grill your protein. Vegetables are easy; you can buy them whole or even precut if you want to save time. Take a bag of lettuce and some precut lettuce, throw it in a bowl, toss it with olive oil and vinegar. You're done!

**Q** **I've seen some weight-loss systems that seem to promise more dramatic losses with less work than Formula 50 does. Why is that?**

**A** Formula 50 isn't intended to be an overnight cure for being out of shape. No such cure even exists. Instead, my program is designed to systematically reprogram your lifestyle from one that may not be the healthiest or fittest to one that will make you feel good and look good. *Lifestyle* is the key word here. When you finish Formula 50, you should want to keep living this way.

Extreme plans bring with them a certain allure, but they're filled with pitfalls. Their marketers prey on your desire for a quick fix to a problem that's been long in the making. It reminds me of the guy who neglects his engine for a hundred thousand miles and then grabs a can of engine sealer at the convenience store when the engine starts banging and hissing. It's not that easy to undo the damage.

My workouts and diets will kick-start your fat loss. Your progress should continue from there at a nice pace. You'll find that there's great satisfaction in achieving steady progress doing this the right way. What's more, your chances of succeeding will skyrocket if you take it slow and steady.

**Q** **I'm doing so many things wrong when it comes to my health and fitness that I become overwhelmed and depressed easily. What should I do to change my thinking?**

**A** Start by obsessing over the things that you're doing right and well, as a means of changing your negative mind-set. Not that you shouldn't take heed of your weaknesses and shortcomings—how else will you improve upon them? But realize that the negatives often seem amplified and dramatic relative to reality, whereas the positives can seem muted and indistinct. The mind is funny that way.

One of the more dangerous traps awaiting you where fitness is concerned is perfectionism. Trust me, you will never do a single set or workout that is perfect. Once you realize that, you can stop beating yourself up for being less than perfect and instead come to view all your fitness efforts in terms of progress, improvement, advancement—words that are relative rather than absolute.

**Q I've tried before and failed. Why will this be any different?**

**A** Because this time, you have my program to follow! I'm only partially kidding. I do think it's essential to follow the right program, one that's been designed by leading experts, based on the latest scientific research, and tested in the gym. My program has been put to the test, and it works, big-time. I won't ask you to do anything you can't handle. Just do it, and you'll experience the results.

Believing in the program is essential for long-term success. I designed Formula 50 in concert with one of the top trainers on the planet, Joe Dowdell, CSCS, so you can be certain that if you do what we ask, if you follow this to a T, success will follow. Nothing would be worse than giving it your all and then not achieving the expected results because you put your faith in a bum program. You can have confidence that Formula 50 works when done right. You have my word on that.

**Q I finish the workouts, but I'm so tired later that I can't do anything. Help!**

**A** These workouts are challenging, and there will be times when you feel a little gassed after completing them. You should feel that way; it's by design. However, as you proceed through Formula 50, the post-workout fatigue should gradually diminish, even as the workouts become more intense. Your body is adapting and becoming more fit, which is the primary benefit of getting in shape. These workouts don't just build your "show" muscles; they strengthen your entire body, including the most important muscle of them all, your heart.

Pay very close attention to our recommendations on nutrition in general, but especially post-workout nutrition. After you train, your body slips into recovery mode, and you need to give it the fuel it needs to repair and recover. If you don't, you may feel tired later as a result. But that's avoidable.

**Q Can I eat too much protein?**

**A** One of Dr. Norton's academic advisors did a study to determine at what level, if any, protein intake begins to create health problems. Basically, he couldn't find that threshold. What he found was that within reason, the more protein people consumed, the healthier they were. That's not to suggest that 400 grams would be healthier than

200. Consuming 400 would be overkill. However, those people consuming 200 or 220 grams remained healthy.

Where protein is concerned, you're more likely to be taking in too little, not too much. Your biggest problem where carbs are concerned will likely be taking in too many, not too few. The meal plans in Formula 50 are set up so that you're on the right side of both of these equations.

**Q** **If I don't see gains happening fast, what should I do?**

**A** Stick with the program. Did you fall out of shape in a matter of days? Of course not! Your current less-than-ideal condition probably reflects years of inattention to training and diet. The good news is that you can reverse the damage far faster than you accumulated it, and you will make some progress almost immediately, although some of it won't be immediately visible in the mirror or on the scale. You might be losing fat and gaining muscle at similar rates, which could result in the same reading on the scale that you saw a week or 2 before. But your body is changing internally in the ways that really matter.

**Q** **As a woman, I'm afraid all this lifting is going to make me look like a guy. Is that a legit concern?**

**A** You're not going to end up looking like a man. The female body doesn't contain the levels of hormones, like testosterone, that the male body does. As a result, gaining muscle is a slower process for women. What your body will do naturally is going to be beautiful. You are going to be strong. Tasks that you now have to ask for help to complete you'll be able to do for yourself. You're going to love how you look. Guys, including me, will think it's sexy.

**Q** **What do you think of yoga?**

**A** Yoga is a form of "active static" stretching. You assume a static position, but you're actively moving into it and engaging many different muscles as opposed to one. Yoga offers many benefits, but you have to take it easy as well. A lot of people get into yoga for physical fitness, and if you don't move very well, you're going to be drenched after your first yoga class. Take it slowly.

**Q I have type 2 diabetes. Can I still follow the Formula 50 program?**

**A** Exercise and healthy eating are exactly what you need if you have type 2 diabetes. Lack of exercise, poor eating, and the resulting weight gain are probably why you got type 2 in the first place. (Type 1 diabetes is an autoimmune disorder, not a lifestyle disease like type 2.)

A multicenter clinical trial called the Diabetes Prevention Program found that lifestyle change (exercise, nutrition, and weight loss) was twice as effective as the leading diabetes medication at preventing diabetes. No side effects either, unlike the vast majority of prescription medications. If you think about it, no wonder lifestyle change works so well. Lifestyle causes the disease.

If you already have type 2 diabetes, consult with your doctor before embarking upon any workout program, including Formula 50. If he or she doesn't encourage you to exercise, get a second opinion, stat. You may have to take heed of interactions between the medications you're taking and your training sessions and dietary changes. Assuming your type 2 diabetes isn't too far advanced, however, you and your doctor may find that the Formula 50 plan eliminates the need for medication.

**Q I'm too tired to make it to the gym tonight. What should I do?**

**A** I recommend that you still go to the gym, if only to reinforce the positive habits you're trying to develop as part of Formula 50. Maybe it was a bad day at work or you had a brutal week, but you'll actually feel better having gone through the workout, even though it might not feel like it at the time. That doesn't mean you have to be at your all-time best that evening and destroy a bunch of personal records. And don't beat yourself up as a result. But still go. You can always decrease your intensity, maybe by increasing your rest intervals a bit that day or by choosing slightly lighter weights than you otherwise would. It's important to develop and maintain the fitness habit. At least you were there and you did what you could do.

**Q I've heard about the thermic effect of food somewhere before, and you talked about it in the diet chapter. So how big an impact does it really have?**

**A** Some experts think the thermic effect constitutes a very large part of your daily energy expenditure, anywhere from 20 to 30 percent. Others peg that figure much lower. One interesting note: Ectomorphs, people with naturally slim body types, tend to have an accelerated thermic effect of food when they eat. You've probably seen these people. When they eat, they actually start sweating.

**Q Aside from stretching and massage, any other recovery techniques I should know about?**

**A** I'll drop two on you. These are more advanced ways to manipulate tissue and enhance performance. This isn't like walking onto a cruise ship and getting a massage.

Active release technique, aka ART, typically isolates parts of the body that need work. The shoulder is the number one area of the body that is injured by people who are into fitness and exercise and working out. The hip structure is another key area. ART can be extremely beneficial and it is a fantastic technique.

PNF (short for proprioceptive neuromuscular facilitation) is a stretching technique that came from the field of physical therapy. The concept is to contract one muscle and then stretch its opposing muscle during that contraction. The muscle being stretched undergoes a bit of neurological release because of the opposing contraction. For example, while your quad is contracted, you might be able to stretch that hamstring more than you otherwise could.

PNF is sometimes done with a personal trainer or a partner, although it could also be done solo with a rope, for example. You'd be flat on your back and then you'd raise one leg with the rope wrapped under your shoe. You could then gently draw the leg forward as far as you could, contract the quad, and then pull it a little closer, increasing the stretch on that hamstring.

**Q I see a lot of people together at the gym. They alternate sets, help each other when the weight gets too heavy, and so on. Should I be doing that as well?**

**A** It's up to you. I know some people who would never go to the gym if they didn't have company, whether that was their trainer or simply a training partner. I also know people who only train alone, and do so by choice. A famous bodybuilder from the 1960s, Dave "The Blond Bomber" Draper, was that way. "I like the company I keep when I'm alone," he has said, referencing his desire to push the iron by himself.

I'm sort of the same way. I don't want to be waiting on anyone. I don't want to be depending on anyone. I don't want to hear about the fight my training partner had with his girlfriend last night, and I don't want to have to coordinate with anyone regarding that day's workouts. I want to walk in and do what feels right to me, depending on my energy that day.

Training in tandem definitely has some advantages. It helps many people stay accountable. They show up because they know their friend is going to show up. That's what's known as *extrinsic* motivation: It comes from outside oneself. That tends to push you in a certain direction. Like a doctor saying, "If you don't start working out, look out, man, a heart attack is coming!"

*Intrinsic* motivation is wanting to show up because it's fun, because you feel better when you do, and because you want the benefits. It comes from within and has a gravitational pull. It's okay to be extrinsically motivated at first, but the longer-term goal is to become intrinsically motivated. At that point, you'll go to the health club because you want to go, and not just because someone else is expecting you.

If you do choose a partner, find someone who's more or less at your level. Training with someone who's raw doesn't do much for you, and training with someone more advanced than you are can also backfire. If you can't do what they do, who do you think gets the better workout? The person who's in worse shape maxes out before he realizes that he went too hard trying to keep up with someone who's more advanced than he is.

**Q Any advice on picking a personal trainer?**

**A** Obviously pick someone well qualified, and someone whom you like hanging out with and taking instructions from. Don't be afraid to go against the grain either. Guys, sometimes it's cool to have a female trainer. I've seen female trainers who will bark something at a client like, "Don't be a pussy, let's go!" You hear that and you're like, *Oh shit!* You say that to me and I'm going to go as hard as possible, until I drop. I'm going to get the most out of that session that I possibly can.

**Q When I started training, I thought for sure my family would support me, but they're often critical, like when they go out for pizza and I opt for healthier fare, like a salad with chicken. How do I deal with this lack of support?**

**A** You would think everyone would be behind you when you start taking back control of your body and trying to lead a healthier life. If they care about you, why wouldn't they, right? As you're finding out, that's not always the case.

So what do you do when you've started out and, instead of supporting you, friends and family seem jealous or envious, practically sabotaging what you're trying to do? You have to really stay focused on your goal or even invite them along. If a spouse is like, "Oh, you're going to the gym *again*," say, "Yeah—why don't you join me?" Try making it inclusive rather than a separate thing that you go off and do by yourself. Convince your friend or partner that you should go to a health club or take a fitness class together. You'll get the support you need, and you might end up saving your loved one's life.

**Q** **I hear a lot of pros and cons about fruit these days. Can I eat it on the Formula 50 program?**

**A** There's a lot of confusion because people have confused high fructose corn syrup (HFCS) with fructose. Slugging down a soda with 50-plus grams of pure sugar is one thing and having a cup of blueberries with 7 grams of fructose and 4 grams of fiber is quite another. Because HCFS sweetens things like soft drinks, we end up consuming way too much of it. Americans are consuming 22 teaspoons of added sugar a day, and HFCS accounts for much of it. That's the problem, not the natural sugar found in fruit, along with vital vitamins and phytochemicals. Fruit? Go for it.

**Q** **So if fruit is good for me, can I just get my fruit servings by drinking orange juice?**

**A** Your question hits at one of the biggest diet traps out there—thinking that fruit and fruit juice are one and the same. Not even. The tall glass of orange juice that looks so good on the breakfast table is really just a glass of bright-colored sugar. The fiber that you would have gotten from the orange has mostly been taken out. If vitamin C is the main reason you're drinking orange juice, just take a vitamin containing it.

This is true of most fruits and their corresponding juices. The three or four apples it takes to make one 8-ounce glass of orange juice contain 12 to 15 grams of fiber—a nice chunk of your recommended daily intake. But that glass of apple juice contains virtually none of that. It's removed in processing.

# 11

# What Happens Next? It's Up to You

**A**S THE FAMOUS SAYING GOES, I NEVER SAID THIS would be easy. I said it would be worth it.

And now here you are. You took charge. You dominated. Now you're enjoying the benefits of increased energy, a better appearance, and higher fitness. You are a new person.

The aftermath of a triumph is always a fresh challenge. *What do I do for an encore?* After all, for the past 6 or even 12 weeks—depending on whether you chose to do both phases of Formula 50 or only one—my program directed your every fitness move. I told you exactly what to do at every workout, what to eat at every meal, and how to rest and recover. I practically told you how and when to tie your shoelaces.

There's no stock answer regarding your next move, no one-size-fits-all plan after The Plan. It depends on your goals moving forward. Maybe you've decided that you want to attempt a triathlon, in which case you would embark on endurance training. Maybe you love how it feels to be leaner and want to continue with that, with the goal of becoming as shredded as a bodybuilder or fitness competitor standing on stage. Maybe you want to keep getting bigger and stronger. Or maybe you just want to continue down the current path of being fitter and healthier, without any specific sports or physique goal.

You can do any of these things. Formula 50 has not only provided you with a foundation but also given you the tools needed to build whatever you want from here. That's why my collaborators and I have spent a lot of time telling you what to do for these 6 to 12 weeks and teaching you about training, nutrition, and the other components of fitness. We want you to take control from here. To paraphrase another famous line, we taught you how to fish.

I do recommend following some sort of program, whether of your own making or someone else's. I think structure proves helpful when it comes to fitness. Now that you're educated, you should be able to judge the worthiness of programs you see in magazines and online. There's a lot of junk out there, but there are also some really smart experts dispensing excellent advice. Especially online, much of this information now comes free of charge.

Your body is telling your brain to keep going, and you should heed that message. Your increased energy and strength can vanish just as quickly as they appeared if you slack off again. What you don't want to do is repeatedly go back to square one and start all over again. That never works well, but it works less and less well as you age.

Don't think in terms of getting "beach-ready," or losing 20 pounds for your wedding, or hitting some other one-time goal. As soon as you do that, you've left the mind-set of making this part of your life and made it something apart instead. In the end, you probably won't stick with it, and I doubt you'll succeed. The process is what you want to master; that's where the real power lies.

I also hope you've reached a point where you no longer fear the things you did before, whether it's the gym environment, criticism from others, muscle soreness, too much muscle, fatigue—you name it. It takes courage to push out of your comfort zone. Just as I left behind the streets, you need to leave behind the couch. I hope you've developed a fearlessness of spirit that now carries over into all the other compartments of your life.

Fearlessness isn't the only quality the program should have developed. Self-reliance, patience, self-confidence—each is forged in the gym every day you train.

Essentially, my team and I took complex training concepts, the kind that used to be available only to high-level athletes, and made them easy for anyone to implement. I hope I've provided some inspiration along the way. I'm well aware that people subconsciously emulate their role models. So I hope that a celebrity who embraces fitness can be a very powerful motivator, a great inspiration. I hope I've been able to serve that function at least in part for you.

Thanks for joining me on this journey.

# Acknowledgments

NO NEW RELEASE EMERGES FROM A VACUUM. WHEN I MAKE A RECORD, THERE MIGHT BE any number of producers working on songs penned by any number of different writers. Various musicians will play on each track, and someone might be singing when I'm not rapping. Behind those creative types is another layer of people offering logistical support, from striking the record deal to signing contracts to making all the arrangements, once the dates and recording studios have been chosen. I may be a solo artist, but every record I make is a team effort.

This book was also a team effort. It involved fewer people than most of my recordings, but it was more collaborative than most books. I'm a recording artist with a passion for fitness that has afforded me a certain depth of information and knowledge; I will admit straight up, however, that I'm not a certified personal trainer, a registered dietitian, a PhD in nutritional sciences, an exercise physiologist, a researcher, or a particularly fast or accurate typist. But those experts and other individuals all inform this work. They were handpicked by me and my coauthor, Jeff O'Connell, to bring my vision to life in *Formula 50*.

My first high five goes to my team at Violator Management, led by Chris Lighty and Laurie Dobbins, Violator's president. Violater represents and supports me across a wide array of business interests and artistic pursuits, so for them to have found time to support me in pursuing a fitness book was no small feat. They had a hand in every aspect of *Formula 50*, and the book wouldn't be what it became without their guidance, encouragement and wisdom.

Sadly, Chris passed away near the end of this project. I still can't believe it. Chris was a good guy, and he will be terribly missed.

I also want to thank my literary agent, Marc Gerald, a vice president at The Agency Group in New York City, for guiding the creation of the proposal and lending support whenever needed. This is my fifth book with Marc, and every one of them has been a new adventure.

My publisher, this go 'round, Avery Books, was a blast to work with from start to finish. Vice President/Editorial Director Megan Newman purchased the proposal and helped guide the book's creation with vision and determination. Editorial Assistant Gabrielle Campo was also indispensable, particularly when it came to helping arrange the photo shoot. Props go as well to Andrea Ho, who served as art director for the cover and also assisted with coordinating the shoot.

My coauthor, Jeff O'Connell, helped work the manuscript with me, sometimes on land, sometimes in the air. Cowriting a book is like cowriting a song, in that two people can take the work to a different place than any one person could have taken it alone. That was certainly the case here.

The actual program (the sets, reps, etc.) was a collaboration among me, Jeff, and Joe Dowdell, a certified strength and conditioning specialist. Together, we took my workout approach and tweaked it for widespread application to a mass audience. Joe is one of the top trainers in the country, and his gym, Peak Performance in New York City, has been ranked among America's ten best gyms by *Men's Health* magazine. We shot the book at Peak, with Joe on hand to ensure that every exercise photo showcased bulletproof form. So you can be sure that you're getting the best information possible in those workout shots and descriptions.

I also want to give a shout to Kindra Hanson, the general manager at Peak, for helping us make those arrangements.

The man behind the camera for the photo shoot was Pavel Ythjall. Special thanks to Pavel and the crew at Pavel Ythjall Photography. Great work. Consider me impressed.

The girl in front of the camera was Rachel DelaCalzada. Thank you for your contribution.

Nutrition is a complicated beast, so I enlisted the best to slay its complexities and turn my personal preferences into this plan. Layne Norton, PhD, holder of a doctorate in nutritional sciences from University of Illinois, worked with me on a scientific approach to eating healthfully as opposed to "dieting." Stephanie M. C. Wilson, MS, RD, CISSN, LDN, the head of nutrition at IMG Academies, came up with meal plans that matched the approach I forged in consultation with Layne.

While Joe, Layne, and Stephanie made the largest contributions of time and expertise, a number of other experts were similarly generous in agreeing to interviews. I'd like to thank them all while singling out two as having been particularly insightful: Perry Nickelston, DC, FMS, SFMA, the director and owner of Stop Chasing Pain and Fitness 201; and Brad Schoenfeld, MSC, master of science in exercise science, a certified strength and conditioning specialist, and a lecturer in exercise science at Lehman College.

Research was handled by Jerilyn Covert, and the transcribing of interviews was done by Tiffiny Trentalange. Special thanks to both young ladies.

Finally, I'd like to recognize the great influence my fans have had on my fitness over the years. Whether I've been gearing up for a video, tour, or movie, they've been the ones inspiring me to reach new heights with my body and mind. So it seems only fitting that I offer this fitness book to them, as an acknowledgment of my gratitude.

# Index